CHAKRA
WORKBOOK

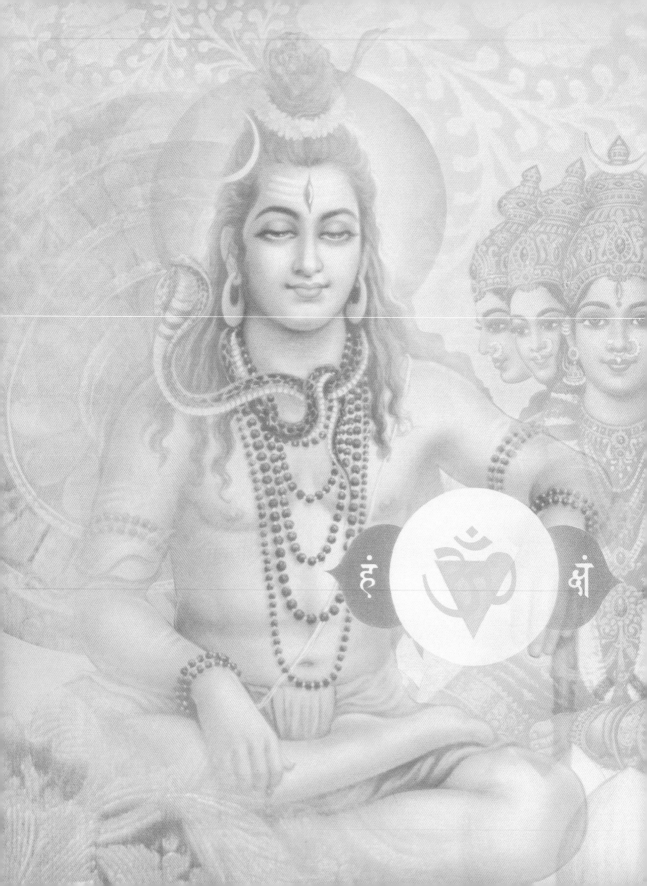

CHAKRA
WORKBOOK

Rebalance your body's vital energies

PAULINE WILLS

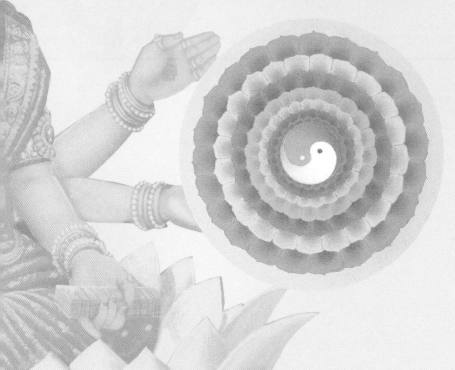

JOURNEY EDITIONS
Tokyo • Rutland, Vermont • Singapore

PLEASE NOTE
The author, packager and publisher cannot accept any responsibility for misadventure
resulting from the practice of any of the principles and techniques set out in this book.
This book is not intended as guidance for the treatment of serious health problems; please
refer to a medical professional if you are in any doubt about any aspect of your condition.

First published in the United States in 2002 by Journey Editions,
an imprint of Periplus Editions (HK) Ltd., with editorial offices at
364 Innovation Drive, North Clarendon, Vermont 05759

Library of Congress Catalog Card Number: 2002104800

ISBN: 978-1-582900-64-3

Distributed by
North America,
Latin America & Europe
Tuttle Publishing
Distribution Center
Airport Industrial Park
364 Innovation Drive
North Clarendon,
VT 05759-9436
Tel: (802) 773-8930
Tel: (800) 526-2778
Fax: (802) 773-6993
www.tuttlepublishing.com

First edition
08   10 9 8 7 6 5 4

AN EDDISON•SADD EDITION
Edited, designed and produced by Eddison Sadd Editions Limited
St Chad's House
148 King's Cross Road
London WC1X 9DH

Phototypeset in Aldus and Barbedor using QuarkXPress on Apple Macintosh
Printed in Singapore

Contents

Introduction

This book describes and explains how you can work with and balance the seven major chakras or 'spinning wheels' of energy in the body. I first discovered the chakra system through my practice of yoga. I was very fortunate to find an Indian teacher who, I later learnt, had devoted most of his life to the study and practice of yoga. He not only taught us the classical postures of yoga (*asanas*) and breathing exercises (*pranayama*), some of which are described in this book, but also introduced us to the spiritual aspect of yoga laid down by the Eastern sage Patanjali. Included with this was information on the aura and chakra system. At the time this fascinated me but also provoked an element of disbelief. I had been brought up in the Christian faith and was still attending and working for the church; therefore any teachings that did not comply with the church's dogma were definitely suspect to me. When I reflect back I laugh at my narrow-mindedness and rigidity and am so grateful that I was gently encouraged to remove my blinkers of conditioning.

Although no longer a church-goer, I still believe that Christ was a realized being alongside other realized beings such as the Buddha and Paramahansa Yogananda. I believe that all religions lead to the ultimate reality of God consciousness and people should choose to follow whichever religion is right for them. Truth is not solely Hindu nor Muslim, Buddhist nor Christian. The follower of truth walks on the path of light, peace, wisdom, power and bliss. The philosophy and practices of yoga are a discipline without dogma and based on truth, and can therefore embrace all religions.

THE ETERNAL TRUTHS

It is believed that the truths contained in all religions are derived from the *Vedas*, the oldest books upon which the Hindu religion is based. The word *veda* means 'knowledge', and when applied to scripture it signifies a book of knowledge. The Vedas are the eternal truths revealed by God to the great Rishis, or seers, of India. It is from the

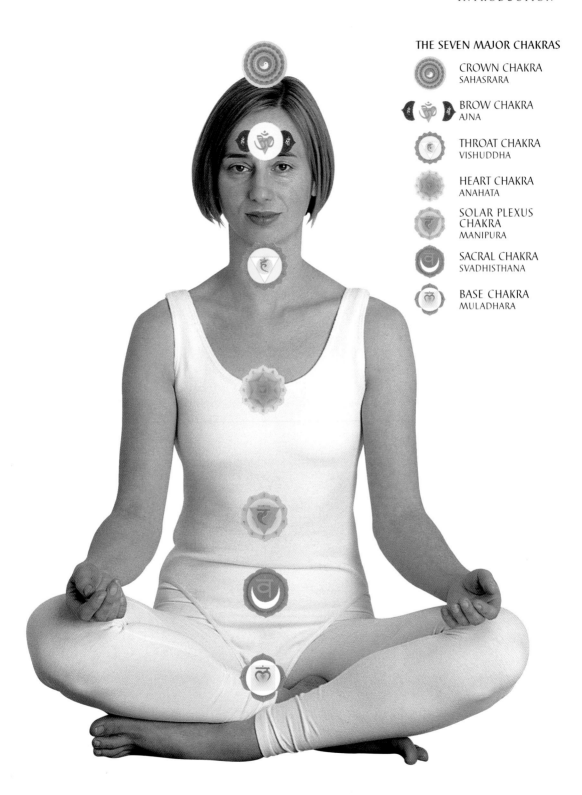

THE SEVEN MAJOR CHAKRAS

CROWN CHAKRA
SAHASRARA

BROW CHAKRA
AJNA

THROAT CHAKRA
VISHUDDHA

HEART CHAKRA
ANAHATA

SOLAR PLEXUS
CHAKRA
MANIPURA

SACRAL CHAKRA
SVADHISTHANA

BASE CHAKRA
MULADHARA

Vedas that our knowledge of yoga comes. The Vedas are divided into books, one of which, the *Upanishads*, contains the essence of the Vedas and is therefore the most important portion. The Upanishads speak of the identity of the individual soul and the Supreme soul and they reveal the most subtle and deep spiritual truths. There are many gods in the Hindu religion, each of which is connected with certain qualities and associated with symbolic animals and icons.

Over time, I have continued to work with yoga. By incorporating visualization, colour and meditation into my practice I gradually realized the importance of the 'subtle anatomy' and chakra system. This system has been used for thousands of years in the East and is now becoming increasingly recognized by Western societies, turning away from the scientific view of health and the body. Each chakra is believed to be a spinning wheel of energy: chakra means 'spinning wheel' in Sanskrit, where the prana, or life-force, of the body is held and organized. Chakras represent a link between the spiritual and the physical, and each one is linked to particular characteristics and parts of the body. When energy is blocked or unbalanced in the body it can affect all areas of life, and by working on the chakras in the ways described in this book, we can promote good health and balance and seek enlightenment.

The aim of this book is to describe the many aspects of the seven generally accepted major chakras, and to outline different ways of working with them to help broaden your understanding, increase your vitality and help you to reconnect with your divine light. Each chakra has a chapter devoted to it. This includes an explanation of the symbolism surrounding the Hindu deities and animals connected with that chakra (such as Sadasiva, left, associated with Vishuddha); the chakra's link with your physical body through the endocrine system, with breathing and visualization exercises to help you locate and sense each chakra, both on the physical body and as reflexology points on either the hands or feet; the associated element and colour; yoga postures or asanas that can be used to clear and activate the chakra; breathing exercises working with the chakra's mantra or sound; meditations on the yantra, or

Sadasiva, the half-man half-woman, is associated with Vishuddha chakra and represents both Shiva and his shakti, or female aspect.

8

geometric form, found within each chakra. The last two chapters, on the Ajna and Sahasrara chakras, vary slightly because they are not associated with a particular element or mantra.

THE AURA AND THE NADIS

The aura, which surrounds and interpenetrates with the physical body, is composed of several layers, or 'sheaths'. Each of these layers is slightly larger than its predecessor, interpenetrates it and extends approximately five centimetres beyond it. It has been suggested that each layer contains its own chakra system, but there is no evidence yet to support this. The chakra system which this book explores is found in the auric layer nearest to the physical body and is known as the 'etheric sheath'. As all the other layers of the aura interpenetrate with this layer, they are affected by the chakras that lie within it.

The etheric sheath is filled with thousands of narrow energy channels, called *nadis*, through which prana flows (these can be likened to the meridians of the Chinese health system). Prana is the life-force derived from the sun, which is essential to all life. On a bright, sunny day prana is abundant and can be seen in the atmosphere as minute particles of brilliant white light. When prana is absorbed into the etheric sheath, it is refracted into the seven spectral colours and the vibrational energy of each colour is absorbed into the chakra that vibrates to its frequency. It is through this extensive net-work of subtle channels that the chakras are connected to the physical body. If the nadis become blocked with stagnant energy that has accumulated from negative thoughts and emotions or from eating too much de-vitalized food, the physical body becomes deprived of energy. If this is not rectified, it will ultimately manifest as a physical disease.

There are thousands of nadis in the body containing the prana or life-force. The major chakras are found where twenty-one nadis intersect.

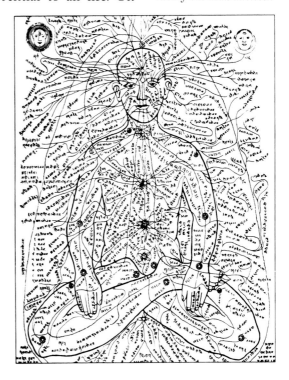

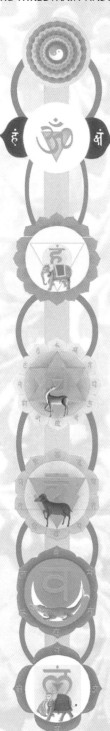

THE THREE MAIN NADIS

I look upon the physical body as a mirror that reflects the condition of all the other aspects of the self. Our spiritual self is reflected in our eyes; our emotional and mental states are shown through skin tone, facial expression and body posture; all three are reflected in the diseases suffered by the physical body.

THE THREE MAIN NADIS

There are three main nadis among the thousands of nadis encompassed in the etheric sheath: the Sushumna, the Ida and the Pingala. The Sushumna Nadi is situated inside the spinal column and is the main channel for the flow of nervous energy. It extends from the Base chakra to the Brow chakra and passes through the four major chakras between (*left*). In the Sushumna are two additional nadis, Vajra and Chitrini. These are enclosed within one another, and it is the 'tube' within the finest of these that is the conduit for the kundalini energy. It is from the Sushumna Nadi that the thousands of minor nadis branch out and link with the nervous system of the physical body.

The Ida Nadi is situated on the left side of the body and the Pingala on the right. Both extend from the Base chakra and intertwine with the major chakras and the Sushumna in a serpentine pattern to their point of termination, the Brow chakra. Ida is associated with coolness, the moon, the right hemisphere of the brain and the parasympathetic nervous system, responsible for relaxation. Pingala is linked with the sun, heat, the left hemisphere of the brain and the sympathetic nervous system, responsible for stimulation. Ida and Pingala receive their supply of prana through the process of respiration and are connected to the left and right nostril respectively. Yogis have taught that when the right nostril is dominant it is time to eat and partake in active work, and when the left nostril is active you should rest, sleep or pursue creative hobbies.

In the etheric sheath of the aura, a major chakra is formed where twenty-one nadis intersect and a minor chakra where fourteen nadis cross. The intersection of the twenty-one nadis in the formation of a major chakra is similar to a ganglion, or plexus of nerve endings, in the physical body. The minor chakras are numerous, with some better known than others. The generally accepted number of major chakras is twelve, from which seven are most commonly recognized and worked with. Five of these seven are situated in line with the physical spine and two are connected to the skull. These are the seven chakras that this book concentrates on. In the twelve-chakra system, there are a further two in the aura above the head, one in the skull, one at the navel and one below the feet.

THE AROUSAL OF KUNDALINI

The ultimate aim of all chakra work is the arousal of kundalini. Kundalini is depicted in the form of a snake which slumbers at the base of the Sushumna nadi. Raising your kundalini, or realizing your full potential, is achieved through will- and mind-power accompanied by appropriate physical action. When aroused, kundalini rises through the aperture hitherto closed by her own coils, up the Sushumna to her spouse, Shiva. On her journey she pierces each of the lotuses or chakras, which turn their heads upwards as she passes through. On reaching the Crown chakra – the thousand-petalled lotus – she brings enlightenment, or 'God consciousness', to the aspirant. When first aroused, kundalini may stay for a very short time at the Crown centre before making her return journey to the Base chakra, but with each arousal the length of her stay increases. Kundalini is sometimes described as the individual bodily representation of the great cosmic power which creates and sustains the universe. Because each human being is a microcosm of that macrocosm, that power also sustains us.

MEDITATION AND BREATHING

Meditation is used throughout this book to bring you awareness of the chakras and the way they influence each other and your body. If you have not meditated before there are a few simple steps you should take before starting. Find a quiet place where you feel comfortable and will not be interrupted. It helps, if you mean to practise regularly, to set aside the same period every day, even if it is only ten minutes first thing in the morning or late at night.

At the heart of our work with yoga and with the subtle energies is meditation, which can take many forms. One form, whose aim is to cleanse and activate the nadis and the chakras in order to bring the whole of the energy system into balance, stems from laya yoga. When combined with specific *pranayama* (breathing) exercises, a very potent system of preventative medicine is established. To work with this it is essential to work with the mantras, geometric forms and the symbolism present in each of the chakras, as explained in the sections devoted to mantras and yantras.

Each chakra has dominant and sub-dominant sounds associated with it, together making a total of fifty, a number that corresponds to the number of letters and sounds in the Sanskrit alphabet. The origins of Sanskrit are unknown, but it is thought in India to have been divinely given, with each letter and its corresponding sound relating to an aspect of human nature.

The meaning of the Sanskrit word 'mantra' is 'the thought that liberates and protects'. The reciting of these words or sounds has the ability to change the consciousness of the reciter. It is believed that all sounds, including our everyday language, create an energy that can be beneficial or detrimental. This is one of the reasons why some monasteries and convents practise the rule of silence, allowing conversation only when it is necessary, during restricted periods. In Hinduism there are literally thousands of mantras grouped according to their purpose or intention. Some are designed to resonate with and activate the chakras; others are used to work with the 'siddhas' or powers that lie latent in each one of us.

One of the aims of laya yoga is to raise the latent energy force (the kundalini) residing in the Base chakra. But its practice also generates a restorative calm within the spinal column and chakras that will then radiate a healing force to the physical organs and endocrine glands connected with each chakra. The aim of this book is to enable you to restore the chakras to balance in order to bring the physical

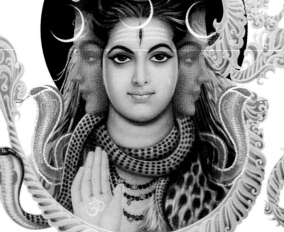

A three-headed representation of Shiva.

body to optimum health and to awaken one's spirituality. Those seeking enlightenment, wishing to work more in-depth with their kundalini, should work with a teacher in addition to the book. The realization of laya yoga's healing and restorative power prompted its use in Ayurvedic medicine. Many of the Ayurvedic doctors were themselves advanced yogis who started to experiment with this subtle energy system. The whole system is fascinating and stimulating in its richness of imagery, and great benefit can be derived by those who practise on a regular basis.

REGULAR PRACTICE

Like the many ways that teach self-growth and empowerment, learning to acknowledge and work with the chakra system takes time, practice and patience, as I myself discovered when walking this path. Working to activate your chakras through asanas necessitates the correct positioning of the body and holding the asana for as long as possible. The postures included in this book are given to help you experience their effect upon your chakras. If you feel that you need more posture work, find your local yoga class and ask if chakra work is included in their curriculum. If you are unfamiliar with yoga, the following pages (*pages 14–15*) are designed to give guidance on some of the most basic postures. These will enable you to attempt the asanas given in later chapters and will be referred back to. It is recommended that you read through all the instructions given before attempting these postures.

I would advise you to read the book right through before trying any of the exercises. This will give you a good foundation upon which to start your exploratory work. If possible, put aside a set time each day for practice in a place that is quiet and free from disturbance. Do not become disheartened if you initially feel that no progress is being made. Progress frequently takes the form of very subtle changes that are not initially detected. If you have chosen to work with this book, I hope that it brings you great joy and a step nearer to understanding and realizing your true self, the ultimate aim of the great journey of life.

BASIC YOGA POSTURES

If you are unfamiliar with yoga, read through these pages before working with the postures given in each chapter that follows in the book. The asanas given here are some of the most basic and are often used as a starting point for other postures. You may wish to refer back to these pages when working on your chakras.

A warm, well-ventilated room is ideal for your yoga sessions. Before you begin, allow a minimum of four hours to lapse from your last meal. The first law of yoga is non-violence and this applies to your physical body too. If yoga is practised on a full stomach, it may interfere with the digestive process, causing physical discomfort. Early in the morning or last thing at night may be the best time and allow you to keep regular hours of practice.

When practising yoga, wear loose or stretchy clothing and use a yoga mat if you have one, or a blanket. Practise in bare feet and remove any jewellery which may hinder movement. Breathing deeply and evenly throughout, hold each posture for as long as feels comfortable to you and never force yourself into any position you find painful. As you practise, you will find your body becoming more flexible and will be able to hold postures for longer.

SUKHASANA
EASY POSTURE

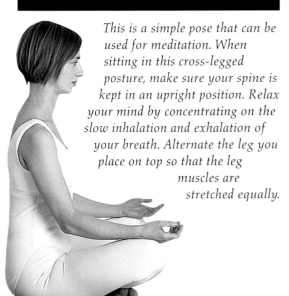

This is a simple pose that can be used for meditation. When sitting in this cross-legged posture, make sure your spine is kept in an upright position. Relax your mind by concentrating on the slow inhalation and exhalation of your breath. Alternate the leg you place on top so that the leg muscles are stretched equally.

ARDHASANA
HALF-LOTUS POSTURE

Bend the left knee and place the left foot against your inner right thigh. Bend the right knee and take the right leg over the left leg, placing the heel of the right foot against the left groin. Work with this posture until you can touch the floor with both knees, then you can attempt the full lotus position.

PADMASANA
LOTUS POSITION

Begin by sitting on the ground with your legs stretched out in front of you. Bend your right knee and place the heel of your right foot against your left groin. Now bend the left knee and lift the leg over the right leg, placing your left heel against your right groin. If your knees do not touch the floor, support them with a wooden or foam block. Alternate the leg you place on top so that both legs become flexible.

SHANKHASANA
CHILD'S POSE

Sitting back on your heels, slowly lower the trunk of your body onto your thighs, and place your forehead on the floor. Place a folded towel beneath your forehead if you are unable to touch the ground. Place your arms alongside your body with the palms facing upwards. Use this posture as a counterbalance to backward bends or the headstand.

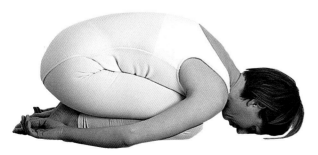

TADASANA
STANDING POSTURE

Standing with your feet hip-distance apart, balance your body weight equally on both feet. Lift your spine, drop your shoulders and extend them back to open your chest. Relax your head and neck muscles, and place your hands by your side. Keep breathing normally.

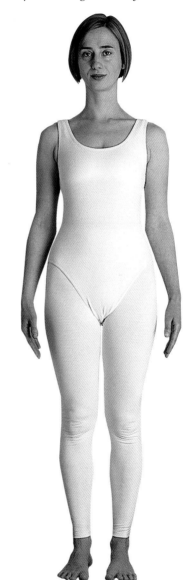

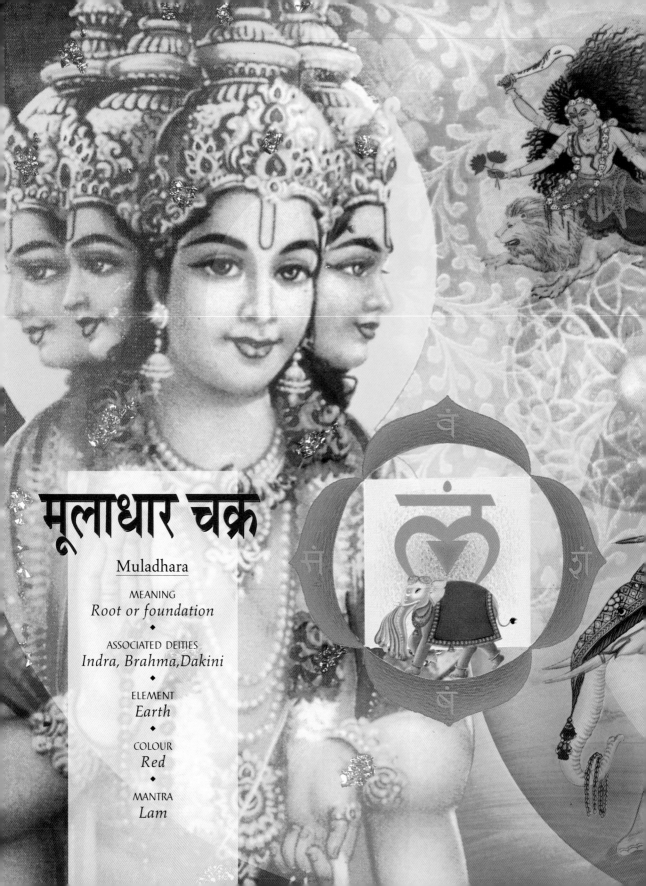

मूलाधार चक्र

Muladhara

MEANING
Root or foundation

◆

ASSOCIATED DEITIES
Indra, Brahma, Dakini

◆

ELEMENT
Earth

◆

COLOUR
Red

◆

MANTRA
Lam

CHAPTER ONE

The Base Chakra

⊷ MULADHARA ⊶

The Base chakra is where we start our journey. The Sanskrit name given to this chakra is Muladhara, meaning root or foundation. This chakra is the foundation upon which we build our lives and it is also the root of the three main nadis, Ida, Pingala and Sushumna, and the root of the kundalini energy. This centre is related to our survival instincts and our feelings of fear and instinct for self-preservation. When our energy is centred in this chakra, fear of being hurt by other people in both a psychological and physical sense may be experienced.

This chakra is depicted as a circle with four outer red petals that have inscribed upon them the Sanksrit letters *va, sa, sa, sa*. By intoning these sacred sounds in a clockwise direction, it is believed that we can experience the four qualities of the four forms of bliss that these petals represent. These are greatest joy, natural pleasure, delight in controlling passion and blissfulness in concentration. In the Indian chakra system the number of petals of any specific lotus is determined by the disposition of the fine, delicate nadis surrounding it. These petals also bear subtle sounds that are produced by the frequency at which they vibrate.

Inside the circle of the chakra lies a yellow square, which is sometimes shown surrounded by eight shining spears. The yellow square represents the earth element and, like the earth, the square shape is solid and stable, making it a perfect foundation upon which to start our spiritual journey.

The spears represent the eight directions of the compass; and when the mantra associated with this chakra is intoned it releases its sound along these eight directions. The spears symbolize the many spiritual paths that lead to the realization of the true self, and also the eight steps of yoga laid down by the sage Patanjali. These steps lead to *samadhi* or enlightenment.

INDRA

Inside the square is Indra *(shown on page 17)*, the deity representing the earth element and the mantra 'Lam'. Depicted in shining yellow he sits on the back of Airavata, king of the elephants. In this depiction Indra has four arms and holds a thunderbolt and normally one dagger. He is the god of warriors but also the god of nature. He reigns in the sky and triumphs in the storm when he thunders and lets loose the rain.

THE ELEPHANT AIRAVATA

The elephant Airavata symbolizes strength, fidelity, long memory, patience and wisdom, but an elephant is a very slow and heavy animal, attributes that portray some of the qualities of this chakra. The skin of the elephant is a soft grey and he is sometimes portrayed with seven trunks – the number relating to the universe, to completeness and totality. In this context the seven trunks represent the seven colours of the spectrum and the chakra to which each of these colours is linked; with the eight notes in an octave; the seven major planets and with the seven constituents that make up the human body. These are earth (*Raja*), fluids (*Rasa*), blood (*Rakta*), flesh, nerve fibres and tissue (*Mansa*), fat (*Medba*), bone (*Asthi*) and bone marrow (*Majjan*). They also link with our desire for security, procreation, longevity, sharing, knowledge, self-realization and union. When all of these attributes are balanced we become complete.

THE GOD BRAHMA

Enclosed in the arm of the mantra 'Lam' is the child creator, Brahma *(shown here in the background)*. Brahma is the first person of the Hindu Trinity and is essentially a creative god and the father of gods and men. He is shown here as red with four faces, each of which is thought to represent one of the four *Vedas*, the sacred scriptures of the Hindus. He has three arms in which he holds the staff, gourd and rosary beads, and a fourth makes a gesture, or *mudra*, which dispels fear.

In Hinduism, the three combined sticks of the staff represent the three gunas which proceeded from the Godhead. These three gunas are: *Sattva*, the light that reveals the true self; *Rajas*, passion, and activity and one's wish for pleasure and wealth; and

Tamas, which is ignorance and binds with sloth, laziness and delusion. The staff also stands for thoughts, words and deeds and the conduit for the rising of kundalini.

The gourd, a vase-shaped vessel, is given to remind us that our search into the mystery of life and spirit begins by working with the qualities and attributes of the Base chakra. The symbolic meaning of the rosary when it is laid down to form a circle is wholeness and time, and its 108 beads stand to remind us of our many incarnations into human form. Only when we are able to transcend this chakra can we progress along our chosen path. To do this we have to rise above fear, shown by the gesture made with Brahma's fourth hand.

THE GODDESS DAKINI

The female deity residing in the Base chakra is Dakini (*above*). With her four arms and brilliant red eyes she is purported to carry the revelation of Divine knowledge. Anyone who meditates upon her will be given this knowledge. In one of her hands she carries the spear (or scissors, as here), representing the masculine principle and the life-giving force. The meaning surrounding the staff and human skull is twofold. It is symbolic of the life-force contained in the head, but it also relates to death through vanity. It is meant to remind us of our need to forgo the pleasures of the world to experience true bliss.

In her right hand Dakini carries a sword and a cup filled with wine, or two lotus flowers. The sword represents protection, and the strength to work with our frailties so that we may be rewarded with the nectar of life (*Amrita*), represented by the lotus flowers or the wine.

KNOWLEDGE, WILL AND ACTION

At the centre of the square is the luminous and soft red down-pointed triangle. This is the yantra, or geometric form, of the lingam and the kundalini which resides within. The downward pointing triangle contains the power of knowledge, will and action; it represents the Ida, Pingala and Sushumna and our need to integrate body, mind and spirit. The triangle also represents feminine energy, and at the Base chakra it houses the male lingam which is said to have the appearance of molten gold and to be shaped like an unopened leaf bud. Around the lingam the kundalini energy, shown as a lightning-like snake, is coiled three and a half times. With her tail in her mouth, her downward-pointing head covers the entrance to the Sushumna.

ENERGIZING MULADHARA

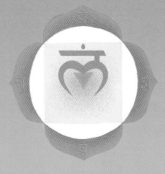

This chakra is our centre of procreation, survival and base instincts and, unlike some of the higher chakras, in the majority of people it is quite vibrant and alive. It influences the blood, spine, nervous system, vagina, legs, testes and the bones.

Each chakra has its opposing tendencies and those of Muladhara are the incoming and outgoing breath. In order to transcend this chakra we must endeavour to rise above our survival instincts. The following exercises will help you to familiarize yourself with the chakra and its energies.

❈ BALANCED ENERGY

When this chakra's energy is balanced it provides vitality for the physical body. It gives a sense of well-being; a feeling of being grounded, centred, sexually affectionate and in control of yourself.

❈ EXCESSIVE ENERGY

Excessive energy here (when the chakra spins too fast) can lead to aggression, make you a domineering, egotist and sexually inhibited.

❈ DEFICIENT ENERGY

Deficient energy here (when the chakra spins too slowly) creates a lack of confidence and depression, accompanied by little will-power to achieve aims in life. It can also cause a loss of interest in sex and a reduced sense of grounding.

❈ PHYSICAL DISORDERS

Some of the physical disorders which may occur when this chakra is not functioning at its full potential are spinal and leg problems, testicular disorders, inhibited rejuvenation of blood cells and haemorrhoids.

AWAKENING MULADHARA ON THE BODY

Sitting in a comfortable position, relax your body before bringing your concentration to the base of your spine, to the Muladhara chakra. Visualize this chakra as a vortex of red energy. Try to feel if the flow of this energy is smooth or jagged. If jagged it suggests accumulated stagnant energy that needs to be cleared.

Bringing your concentration to your feet, breathe in a clear red light from the earth, through the soles of your feet, up your legs and into your Base chakra. As you exhale, imagine this red stream of energy swirling from your chakra, into your aura and back down into the earth. Continue with this exercise for five to ten minutes. At the end of this time, concentrate once more on the chakra and feel for any changes that have taken place.

▶ *This chakra is located at the perineum, between the anus and the genitals, and is also referred to as the root centre. It is associated with the pelvic plexus.*

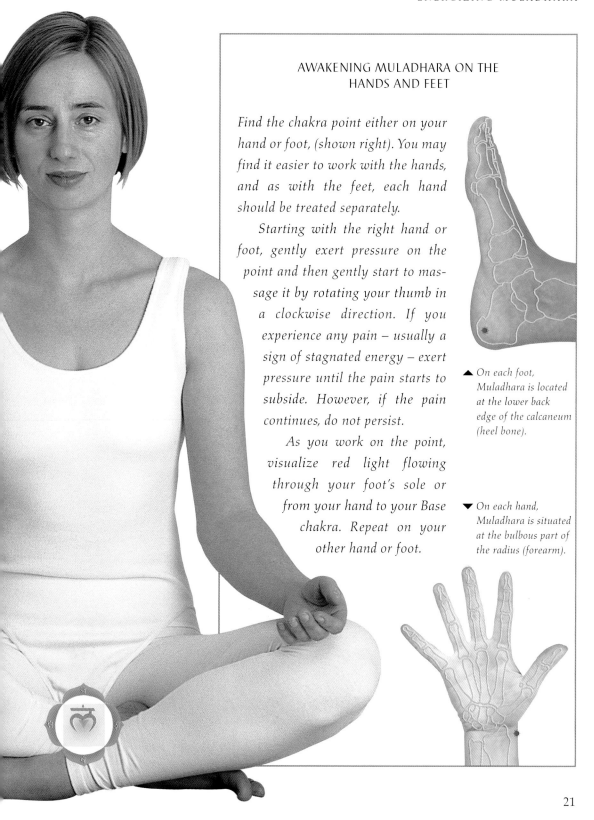

AWAKENING MULADHARA ON THE HANDS AND FEET

Find the chakra point either on your hand or foot, (shown right). You may find it easier to work with the hands, and as with the feet, each hand should be treated separately.

Starting with the right hand or foot, gently exert pressure on the point and then gently start to massage it by rotating your thumb in a clockwise direction. If you experience any pain – usually a sign of stagnated energy – exert pressure until the pain starts to subside. However, if the pain continues, do not persist.

As you work on the point, visualize red light flowing through your foot's sole or from your hand to your Base chakra. Repeat on your other hand or foot.

▲ *On each foot, Muladhara is located at the lower back edge of the calcaneum (heel bone).*

▼ *On each hand, Muladhara is situated at the bulbous part of the radius (forearm).*

THE EARTH ELEMENT

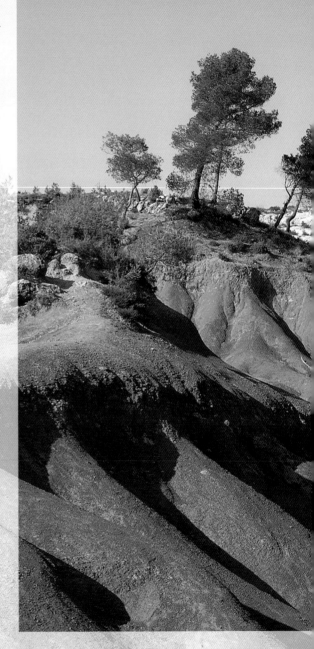

In Indian philosophy the universe is made from a combination of five basic ingredients, each containing different proportions of matter and consciousness. The first of these, the earth element, with its quality of solidity, is associated with Muladhara chakra. It is symbolized by the yellow square of the chakra symbol shown on page 16.

The four sides of this square represent the four corners of the earth and the four elements. Perhaps more importantly, they also denote the four qualities needed when following any spiritual path: honesty, straightforwardness, integrity and morality. Hindus look upon the square as the archetype and pattern of order in the universe. If we are aiming to walk a spiritual path we need an ordered and structured life.

When focusing on this element think of the earth as a living entity who is also trying to make a quantum leap to the next level of consciousness. In order to do this she has to rid herself of the toxins that we have polluted her with. When you work with this element by doing the exercise opposite, try to mentally send love and light into the earth and find ways to help ease pollution.

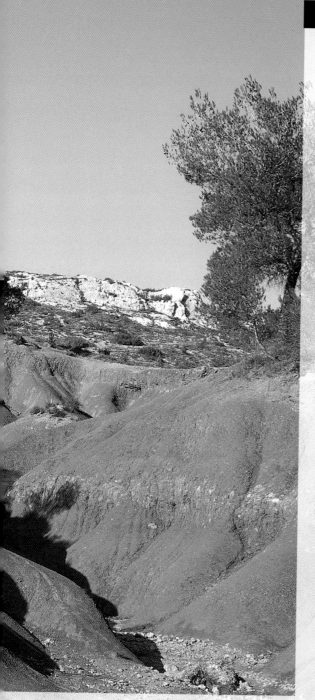

EXERCISE

When working with your chakras it is important to stay grounded. This can be achieved by gardening or growing plants or flowers, or through performing specific exercises, such as the one outlined here, to maintain the energy balance of this chakra.

Ideally this exercise should be performed either standing or sitting with your bare feet on the earth. If you do not have a garden or access to some outside space, sit indoors with your bare feet on the floor.

Start by breathing in and out to a count of five to release any tension in your body and to still your mind. Now, bring your concentration to your feet. Visualize roots extending from the soles of your feet down into mother earth, anchoring you to her. Allow the earth to feed nourishment into your feet, legs and Base chakra through the roots you have laid down. Feel the stabilizing effect this has.

After a few minutes of working with this, shift your concentration to the crown of your head. Visualize a shaft of white energizing light flowing through your head, down your spine, into your legs, feet and through your roots into the earth. Give this vitalizing energy to the earth in return for the nourishment she is giving you.

When you feel ready, withdraw your roots from the earth and contemplate the grounding effect this has had on you.

COLOUR AND VISUALIZATION

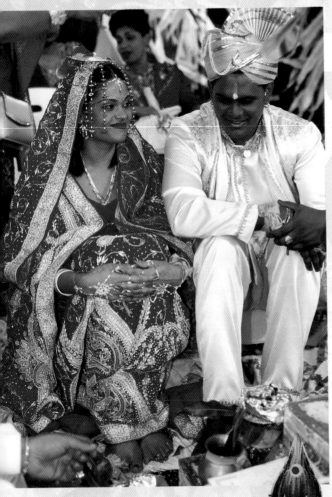

Red, the colour associated with the Base chakra, is worn at Indian weddings as a sign of fertility and procreation. This symbolic gourd, right, is used on auspicious occasions to bring good luck.

The colour red is associated with the Base chakra. Red is a loud colour with low energy. It is connected with sexuality and with the arousal of sexual energy. Its darker shades denote aggressiveness and fear, thought to be the most harmful emotion to our spirit because it prevents us from walking forward. Most fears stem from conditioning, which is something we need to look at and work with if our aim is to become the master of this chakra's energy. Perhaps we need to keep reminding ourselves that what was right for us yesterday may not be right for us today.

The characteristics associated with the four red lotus petals relate to some of the qualities of this chakra. Red is the colour linked with masculine energy, warmth, procreation, survival and rebirth.

RED IN CULTURES AROUND THE WORLD

In India, a bride is adorned in a red sari on her wedding day to symbolize fertility. Red is also deeply bound up with the most important life-events of many of the indigenous peoples of the world. These include the Craho Indian Tribe, Brazil, whose medicine man has his face painted red in ceremonies and whose dead are daubed with red ochre, symbolizing rebirth into the spiritual realm.

ENERGY OF THE BASE CHAKRA

The main preoccupation of those whose energy is centred at the Base chakra is physical survival. For this reason their thoughts may be centred on the fear of being physically or psychologically hurt or they may have a tendency to hurt others. If this centre is deficient in energy, you can become lethargic and deprived of the will-power needed to achieve your aims in life. You could also lack confidence, feel insecure or be filled with anxiety and worry.

You can learn to become the master of this centre's energy through colour visualizations and the other exercises in this chapter. These will enable you to transform any negativity or sluggishness into a strong, positive physical energy. This will reward you with a great love for life, coupled with contentment and inner peace. If you suffer from any complaints in the parts of your body linked with this chakra (*see page 20*) it will be particularly beneficial for you to work with it on a regular basis.

VISUALIZATION WITH RED

S it comfortably in a warm, quiet place. Make sure your spine is straight, your body relaxed and your mind peaceful and quiet.

Bring your concentration to both feet and imagine that they are resting on a bright red carpet. Move your toes to feel the carpet's texture and softness and then try to feel the warmth and energy this colour is sending through the soles of your feet.

Visualize both your feet saturated in red light and imagine this colour travelling from your feet, up your legs into the Base chakra. Quietly contemplate the relationship the colour has with this chakra. Remember that Muladhara is associated with the physical body, with procreation, and that red, its dominant colour, has slow, warm and vibrant attributes.

Focusing on the Base chakra, visualize a clear, vibrant red flowing from this centre into your aura, down both your legs and back to your feet.

Continue to work with this exercise for five to ten minutes. At the end of this time, your legs and feet will feel warm and energized, and you will also experience higher energy levels generally.

STIMULATING ASANAS

The yoga postures (*asanas*) shown here have been chosen as they work directly with the Base chakra. There are other postures that work equally well with this chakra, although space does not permit them to be included here.

In order to stimulate the chakra when working with yoga, it is essential that the body position is correct, and to maximize the effect on the chakra, the posture should be held for as long as is possible, without strain. While holding the postures, breathe deeply and evenly. When working with the Base chakra, visualize a pure, clear, red light radiating from it. Attempt to feel the energy of this colour on and around your coccyx.

It is very tempting to practise the asanas that are easy for you. This is not a good idea as each asana helps strengthen specific parts of the physical body in preparation for the Shakti energy to rise. This only happens when you are spiritually ready.

If you wish to pursue the yogic path, I would recommend that you find an experienced teacher.

WARM-UP ASANA
THE ARM-LEG LINK

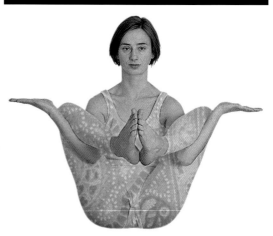

❶ Sit on the floor with your legs stretched out and your spine straight.

❷ Bend your knees, placing the soles of your feet by your buttocks. Your feet should be approximately 15 cm (6 inches) apart.

❸ Take your arms between your legs and under your knees.

❹ Exhaling, recline the trunk of your body slightly backwards to allow you to balance on your buttocks with your feet raised from the floor. Open your knees as far as possible.

❺ Keep your in-breath the same length as your out-breath and visualize the energy of the chakra expanding and contracting in synchronization. Return to the sitting position.

BENEFITS:

This posture stretches the inner thigh muscles, making it a good posture to work with during pregnancy. It aids balance and poise and helps in working towards the full lotus posture.

ARDHA NAVASANA 2
THE BOAT POSTURE

YOGA MUDRASANA
ARM AND SHOULDER STRETCH POSTURE

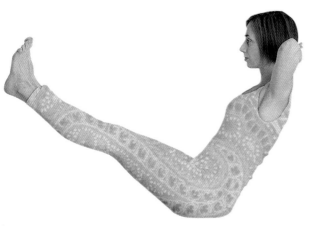

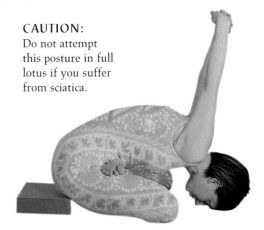

CAUTION:
Do not attempt
this posture in full
lotus if you suffer
from sciatica.

1 *Sit on the floor with your legs outstretched in front of you.*

2 *Keeping your spine straight, interlock your fingers and place them on the back of your head, just above the neck.*

3 *Exhale and recline the trunk back, simultaneously raising your legs from the floor to an angle of 30–35 degrees. Your head should be in line with your feet.*

4 *Hold the posture for approximately thirty seconds while bringing your concentration to the Base chakra and the colour red.*

5 *Exhaling, come back to the sitting position.*

1 *The correct sitting posture for this asana is full lotus position (see page 15). If you are unable to achieve this position, sit either in simple cross-legged posture or in half-lotus posture (see page 14).*

2 *Inhaling, clasp your hands behind your back.*

3 *Exhaling and keeping your spine straight, move the trunk of your body forward from the hips, bringing your chin as near to the floor as possible. At the same time raise your arms upwards.*

BENEFITS:

This asana tones the kidneys, gall bladder, liver and spleen. It works on the thighs and abdominal muscles. It also improves balance, reduces nervous tension and aids digestion.

BENEFITS:

This posture relieves stiffness in the arms and shoulders. It intensifies the peristaltic action, relieving constipation and improving digestion.

BREATH AND SOUND

The breathing exercises given in this book should be practised regularly in a place that is quiet, warm and well-ventilated. Adopt a posture that is comfortable for you. This can be on a straight-backed chair, with both feet resting on the floor and your hands resting on your thighs, or on the floor in a simple cross-legged posture.

When working with the mantras, an intonation of the sounds associated with the chakras, adopt the same sitting posture. With each intonation of the mantra, try to feel the energy created by the sound vibrating in the chakra you are working with. This vibration will help clear stagnant energy and maintain the chakra in a state of balance.

CAUTION
If you become breathless or dizzy when doing these exercises, resume normal breathing. As your body and lungs become used to working with these exercises, any symptoms initially experienced should disappear.

THE RHYTHMIC BREATH

Sit comfortably in one of the positions described on the left. Relax your body and bring your concentration to your breath. Focus on your natural rhythm of breathing for approximately five minutes. This will help quieten your mind and induce a deeper state of relaxation.

When you are ready, breathe in to a count of five and out to a count of five. If you find this difficult, reduce the number of counts to four or three. With practice your lung capacity will increase, enabling you to work up to a count of seven. Concentrate on the top of your nose to feel the change in temperature with your in-breath and out-breath. Try to visualize the passage of air as it enters and leaves your nostrils.

Continue to work with the rhythmic breath for five to ten minutes. When you have completed this, focus on your Base chakra and imagine white light being drawn into it with each inhalation. Visualize this energy as liquid light and when you exhale, envisage it cleansing and restoring this chakra to balance.

MANTRA EXERCISE

After completing the rhythmic breathing exercise, left and above, continue to concentrate on your Base chakra and try out the following mantra exercise.

The Sanskrit mantra for the Base chakra is 'Lam' (pronounce the 'a' as in 'barn'). To work with the mantra, take a deep breath, open your mouth and start to intone the first part of the mantra 'laaa …' before gently bringing your lips together to intone the 'mmm'.

When you run out of breath, take another deep breath and repeat. If you are able, intone the mantra on middle C. Otherwise, make the intonation on the note that feels most comfortable to you. Experiment without feeling self-conscious and you will find the note that works for you.

Keep the sound soft and gentle and try to feel in your body where it is resonating. You may like to experiment with the pitch until you feel the vibration in and around your Base chakra. Concentrate on Muladhara and project the sound there.

Try to continue this exercise for five minutes. The time you are able to focus in this way will gradually increase as you become more experienced. When you have finished, sit quietly and reflect for a few minutes on the way that this exercise has made you feel.

WORKING WITH THE YANTRA

To the lay person, yantras may appear to be little more than interesting designs. However, for the student studying the chakra system, yantras are mystical symbols of higher planes of consciousness. When these are meditated upon in a prescribed manner you become attuned to the vibrations embodied within them. With continued practice your consciousness is drawn to the planes of which the yantras are graphic representations.

Many yantras are universal and are used in meditation by yogis and by those following other esoteric paths. Each yantra imparts its own unique form of energy, illumination and refinement. Regular practice will enable you to become sensitive to the value of a particular yantra as it relates to your personal development.

The yantra for the Base chakra is a yellow square enclosing a red downward-pointing triangle (*see right*). When working with the following exercise, place the drawing in a position where you can see it without strain.

There is no set time for this exercise as you should try to work on it in your own personal way. Try to remain relaxed throughout and focused on the yantra image. You might like to consider recording your experiences in a diary as some students find this beneficial.

EXERCISE

Sitting comfortably in full lotus or cross-legged pose, begin by working with the rhythmic breath exercise (see page 28) for a few minutes to relax your body and mind.

When you are ready, begin your yantra exercise by focusing on the yellow square. This square symbolizes the solidity of the earth and helps you keep both your feet rooted in mother earth. Do you feel that you are grounded and have created for yourself a solid foundation upon which to start your work of self-development? If not, work with the exercise given for the earth element on page 23.

The yellow of the square is related to the intellect and is a colour that will allow you to examine any changes you need to make for self-growth. Initially, working with self-growth involves the use of intellect but with practice you can reach a stage where you are able to transcend the intellect and view your life from a higher perspective. Making the necessary changes then becomes easier because in this state we are able to detach from our physical life.

From the square, move your gaze to the downward-pointing red triangle. This represents the feminine energy, although it houses the male lingam. These two symbols speak of duality and the need to work towards integration and wholeness, which challenges the need to reflect upon our own duality.

Contemplate the masculine and feminine energy that resides in you to see if you are working with both of these equally. Apply the same consideration to the time you allocate for work and pleasure. Carrying out logical tasks uses the left or male hemisphere of your brain and creative pursuits use the right, or female, hemisphere.

Consider your diet. A wholesome diet should contain equal amounts of acidic and alkaline food. Too much of one or the other creates an imbalance which can lead to physical illness. To create wholeness you need to maintain balance in your life.

Experience the effect of polarity through your breath while remaining focused on the yantra. This can be done by working with the rhythmic breath exercise given on page 28. Keeping your inhalations

and exhalations equal in length, you will experience a sense of calmness and peace. Uneven and rapid breathing will create tension within you and you will find yourself unable to consider clearly the yantra and your purpose in focusing on it.

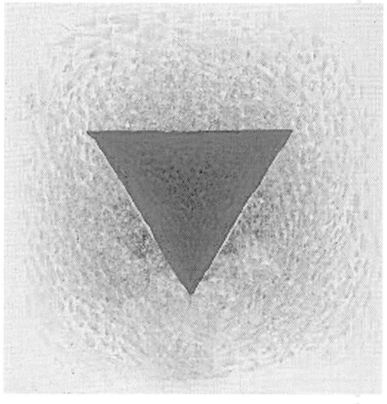

To complete this exercise, contemplate the explanation given for this yantra. Address imbalance in your life and consider changes you feel are necessary for your spiritual growth.

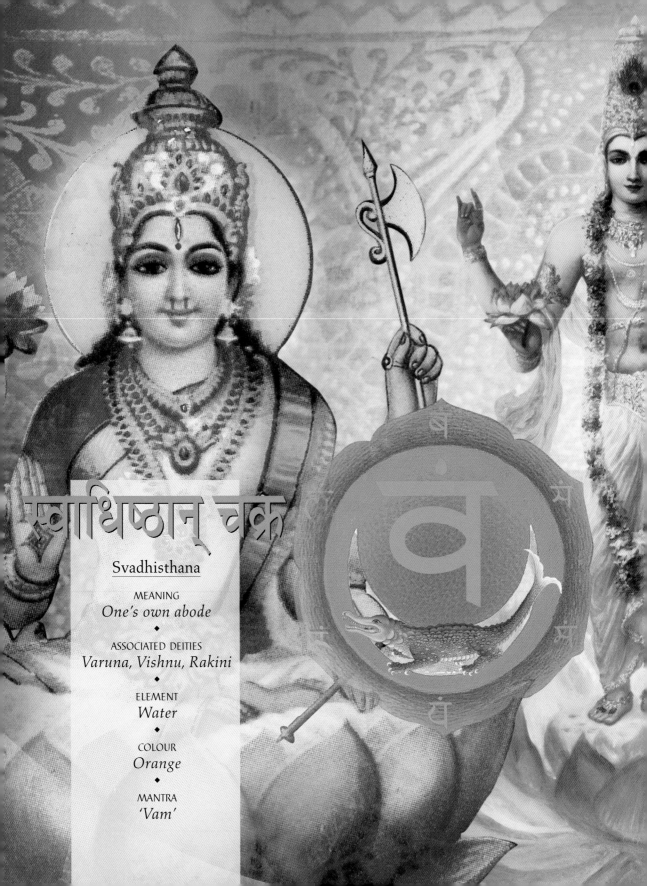

स्वाधिष्ठान् चक्र

Svadhisthana

MEANING
One's own abode

◆

ASSOCIATED DEITIES
Varuna, Vishnu, Rakini

◆

ELEMENT
Water

◆

COLOUR
Orange

◆

MANTRA
'Vam'

CHAPTER TWO

The Sacral Chakra

⟶ SVADHISTHANA ⟵

The Sanskrit name for this chakra is Svadhisthana, meaning 'one's own abode'. Unlike the Base chakra, whose primary concern is for our self-preservation and survival, this chakra is more concerned with pleasure in life. Its relationship with our sexuality has gained it the reputation of being the centre for pleasurable addiction to food, drink and material comforts. Anyone who has their energies focused here will be preoccupied with sensual pleasure and experience.

Svadhisthana is depicted as a circle with six orange outer petals with the letters *ba, bha, ma, ya, ra* and *la* inscribed upon them. The modes of being represented by the letters are affection, pitilessness and all feelings of destructiveness, delusion, disdain and suspicion. The orange petals symbolize this chakra's creative, sexual energy and the joy that comes with the creation of a human form for an incarnating soul.

Inside the circle is a crescent moon, representing the water element. The moon speaks of light, growth and regeneration and its energy controls the ebb and flow of the oceans, the seasons, rainfall and floods as well as our own emotional fluctuations. This chakra comes into play during puberty, a time of great emotional trauma in many young people, and through the moon's influences, the menstrual cycle is affected.

THE GOD VARUNA

Varuna, the deity associated with the water element and the mantra 'vam', is often shown seated within the crescent moon.

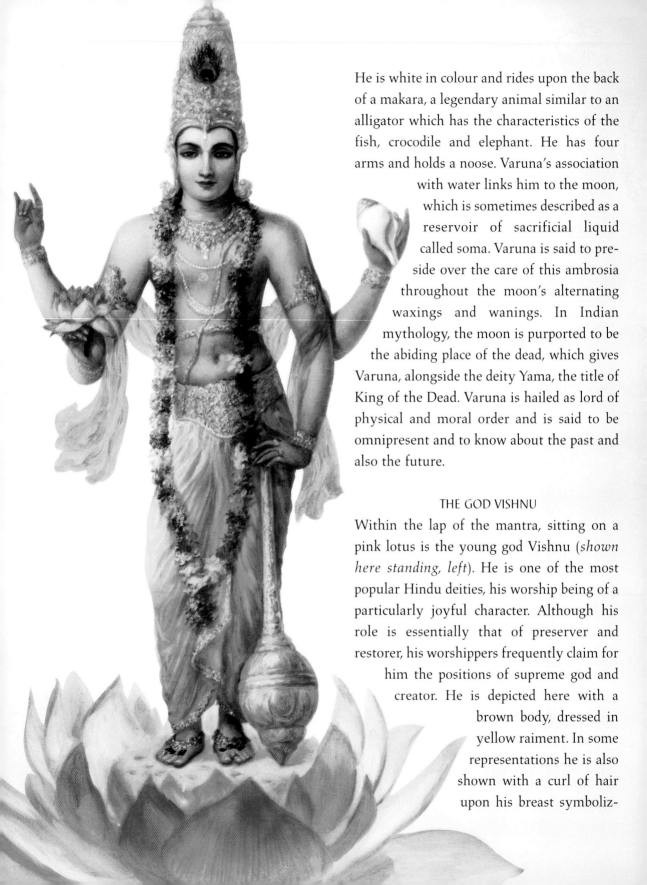

He is white in colour and rides upon the back of a makara, a legendary animal similar to an alligator which has the characteristics of the fish, crocodile and elephant. He has four arms and holds a noose. Varuna's association with water links him to the moon, which is sometimes described as a reservoir of sacrificial liquid called soma. Varuna is said to preside over the care of this ambrosia throughout the moon's alternating waxings and wanings. In Indian mythology, the moon is purported to be the abiding place of the dead, which gives Varuna, alongside the deity Yama, the title of King of the Dead. Varuna is hailed as lord of physical and moral order and is said to be omnipresent and to know about the past and also the future.

THE GOD VISHNU

Within the lap of the mantra, sitting on a pink lotus is the young god Vishnu (*shown here standing, left*). He is one of the most popular Hindu deities, his worship being of a particularly joyful character. Although his role is essentially that of preserver and restorer, his worshippers frequently claim for him the positions of supreme god and creator. He is depicted here with a brown body, dressed in yellow raiment. In some representations he is also shown with a curl of hair upon his breast symbolizing *sattva*, *rajas* and *tamas*, the three qualities of nature which are thought to be the original source of the material world. He wears a large shining gem and a garland extending to his knees. This garland is made with flowers from the four seasons to symbolize the four basic elements. He is shown with four arms. One holds the conch from which the primordial sound of 'aum' is thought to have first issued and which at this chakra represents the feminine principle, the water element, regeneration and fertility. The mace and the lotus remind us of our need to gain mastery over our chakras in order to utilize their power for our own spiritual development. The lotus flower upon which Vishnu stands is his emblem as the god of the sun. Occasionally he is shown with a discus of light, symbolizing the rotation of our chakras.

THE GODDESS RAKINI

Beside Vishnu, sitting on a double lotus and adorned in celestial clothes, is the radiant goddess Rakini *(right)*. Her uplifted arms hold the lotus, the trident and a sharp battle-axe. She is shown with three red eyes and with blood flowing from her nostrils.

The battle-axe and the trident, symbols of the fire god Agni, demonstrate the concept of opposites within this chakra. The chakra's principal element is water, but when this comes into contact with the fire element, the water is changed into vapour which is less dense and therefore able to rise into the atmosphere. This symbolism demonstrates our task of transforming this centre's energies so that they, like the vapour, can rise to bring us to a higher level of consciousness.

FIRE AND WATER

In women this transformation happens naturally during the menopause when the lower creative energies, used to create a body for an incarnating soul, are transmuted to the throat centre where they are used for spiritual pursuits. An interesting theory is that at this time of a woman's life, the fire and water elements alternate in their dominance, and maybe it is this that gives rise to hot flushes and emotional imbalances. It is believed by some that taking hormone replacement therapy binds our lower creative energies to the Sacral chakra, thus preventing their natural transformation.

It is written in ancient Tantric documents that those who work with and meditate upon Svadhisthana are freed from the six passions of lust, anger, greed, delusion, pride and envy. To achieve this state takes many years of regular practice.

ENERGIZING SVADHISTHANA

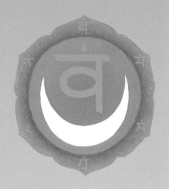

❀ BALANCED ENERGY

When this chakra's energy is balanced you will be in touch with your own emotions, and trusting towards others..

❀ EXCESSIVE ENERGY

Excessive energy here (when the chakra spins too fast) can cause an over-emotional, aggressive, over-ambitious, manipulative nature, over-indulgent and obsessed with sex.

❀ DEFICIENT ENERGY

Deficient energy here (when the chakra spins too slowly) creates feelings of over-sensitivity, timidity, resentment, distrust and guilt.

❀ PHYSICAL DISORDERS

Possible ailments arising from imbalance here include bladder and kidney disorders, circulatory problems, intestinal complaints, shallow and irregular breathing, low energy, disturbances of the central nervous system, migraines and disfunction of the reproductive organs.

This chakra is the source of vitality for the etheric body and governs our love/hate relationships. Its opposing forces are attraction and repulsion, feelings governing desires. To transcend this chakra is to rise above our likes and dislikes in order to see all things as part of the whole. On a physical level this chakra influences the female reproductive organs, the mammary glands, skin, kidneys and the adrenal glands. Unlike the powerful aggressive masculine energy at the Base centre, this centre's energy is gentler but is complementary to the masculine energy. The following exercises will familiarize you with the chakra and its energies.

AWAKENING SVADHISTHANA
ON THE BODY

Start this exercise by slowly inhaling and exhaling to a count of five. Repeat this eight to ten times. Now bring your concentration to the chakra. With the same rhythm of breathing, on your next inhalation visualize a shaft of orange light entering your body through your feet, moving up your legs and entering your Sacral chakra.

As you exhale, visualize this colour radiating from your chakra, into your aura. Continue with this exercise for approximately five to ten minutes. As your concentration deepens, try to feel the Svadhisthana chakra. The feeling you may experience could be one of heat or a gentle vibration. When you feel ready, resume normal breathing.

▶ *On the physical body, Svadhisthana is located halfway between the pubis and the navel.*

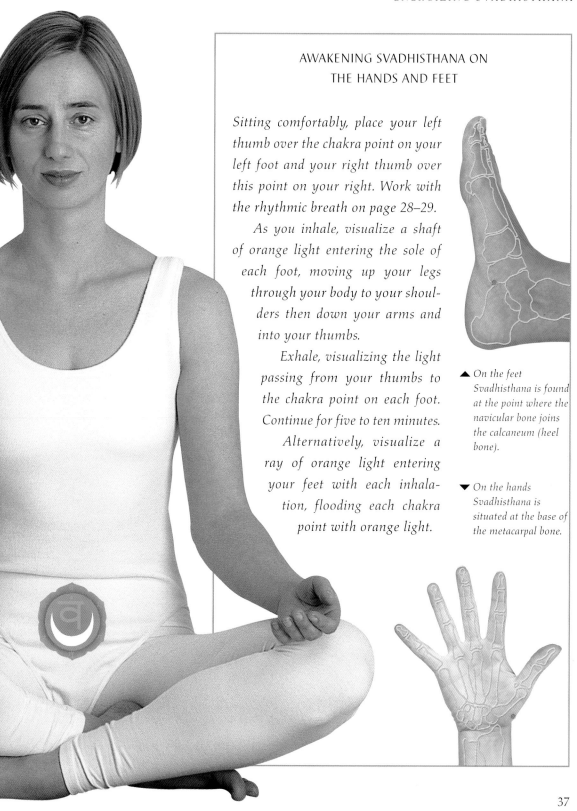

AWAKENING SVADHISTHANA ON THE HANDS AND FEET

Sitting comfortably, place your left thumb over the chakra point on your left foot and your right thumb over this point on your right. Work with the rhythmic breath on page 28–29.

As you inhale, visualize a shaft of orange light entering the sole of each foot, moving up your legs through your body to your shoulders then down your arms and into your thumbs.

Exhale, visualizing the light passing from your thumbs to the chakra point on each foot. Continue for five to ten minutes.

Alternatively, visualize a ray of orange light entering your feet with each inhalation, flooding each chakra point with orange light.

▲ *On the feet Svadhisthana is found at the point where the navicular bone joins the calcaneum (heel bone).*

▼ *On the hands Svadhisthana is situated at the base of the metacarpal bone.*

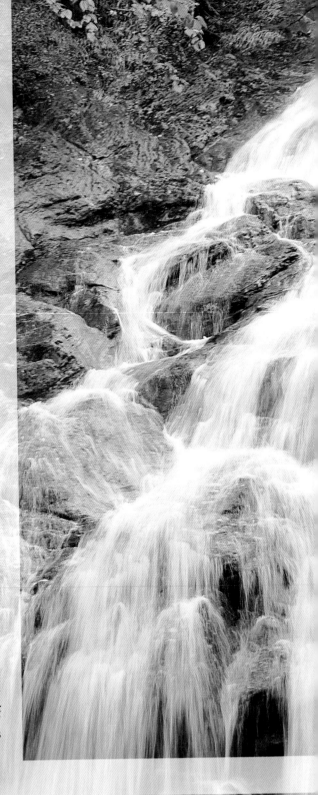

THE WATER ELEMENT

Water, the element related to the Sacral chakra, is essential to life. The rain replenishes the earth for plants and crops, and by filling the rivers and streams, which are linked to the circulatory system of the earth, it sustains all life.

Water, a symbol of life, is also associated with death. Hindus scatter the ashes of loved ones into the sacred river Ganges to gain eternal life. Water is also a medium for healing. Many sick people travel to Lourdes, in France, and Walsingham, in England, to be cured by the sacred water there. In baptism, water is used as a symbol of purification.

The lotus flower is a flower of light and great beauty which thrives in water. It depicts spiritual development, starting life with its roots in mud and silt and growing through the opaque water, eventually flowering in the sun and light.

We too are often submerged in the muddy waters of the mind and the collected debris of past actions but, like the flower, we must rise above our selfish desires and allow our higher consciousness to flower in the light of the spiritual sun. The shining lotus of the spiritual self will appear when the waters have receded and the mud is washed away.

EXERCISE

Visualize yourself at the dawn of a new day, contemplating the bud of a lotus flower resting upon the still waters of a pond. Let your imagination take you to the flower's roots, embedded in the mud at the bottom of the pond. Contemplate your life and the situations and conditioning that prevent you from rising out of the mire of fear and helplessness.

See how the strength of the root allows the lotus to push up through the murky water. There are times when we need this strength to become disentangled from the web of chaos and delusion that we have created. See the flower emerging into the sunlight. At exactly the right moment, the protective covering housing the delicate petals falls away and the flower opens to reveal its great beauty.

Similarly, your spiritual development necessitates the peeling away of protective layers if you are to blossom in the light of the spiritual sun. The petals of the lotus bud can be damaged if it opens prematurely. If you try to develop spiritually too quickly you may also be damaged. Listen to your intuition.

With the passing of dawn, the sun's gentle warming rays encourage the bud of the lotus to open to its full glory. Before ending this meditation, contemplate your own spiritual awakening.

COLOUR AND VISUALIZATION

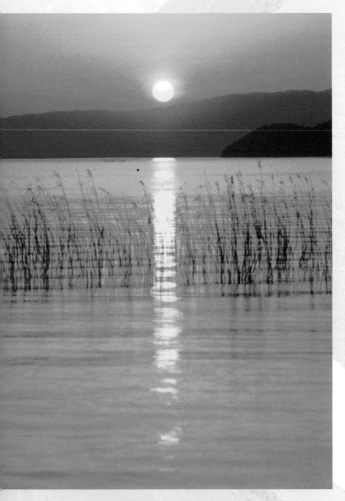

▲ *Orange, the colour linked to the Sacral chakra, is a warm, energizing colour. that has the power to instil joy. Visualizing the sun setting, as in the exercise opposite, can dispel negativity from the past.*

Orange is the colour associated with the Sacral chakra. It is believed that the colour originally gained its name from the Arabic word *naranj*, meaning fruit. The rich, vibrant orange dyes that appeared in the nineteenth century were produced from the red fleshy root of the madder flower. Today's deep, luxurious shades are produced from synthetic dyes.

Orange lies midway between the red and yellow rays in the visible light spectrum, and influences both physical vitality and intellect. Orange, like red, is associated with sexuality but in a much gentler way. Linked with joy and happiness, it gives freedom to our thoughts and feelings by dispersing heaviness and allowing the body its natural, joyful movements. Orange is said to bring about changes in our biochemical structure which can result in the lifting of depression.

Someone who is physically attracted to orange could be lacking in energy, feeling depressed or suffering from a female disorder. Being drawn to it emotionally or mentally may imply a lack of either emotional or mental joy and stimulation. There are many reasons why this may occur. Although orange can temporarily uplift and energize you, a complete cure for the problem suffered can only be found if the cause is acknowledged and worked with. The best person to help you with this is a qualified colour practitioner.

To take in orange, work with visualization, colour breathing (mentally absorbing the colour as you breathe) and wear orange clothes. When working with coloured clothing, white underwear should be worn beneath it, otherwise the colour you receive will be a mixture of the two colours you are wearing. Light therapy is a very effective and powerful way of working with colour, but is best practised by a colour therapist, rather than attempted at home.

Spiritually, this colour challenges us to examine our beliefs. When wearing orange or working with the visualization (*right*) you may find that a strongly-held belief no longer seems true. If this feeling remains strong over a period of time you may consider discarding this belief and searching for your own truth in life.

VISUALIZATION WITH ORANGE

Sitting in a comfortable position with a relaxed body and quiet mind, imagine that you are sitting on a clifftop at sunset, looking across the sea to the horizon. Listen to the waves as they break on the shore, and become aware of their rhythmic pattern. Synchronize your breath with their ebb and flow, inhaling as the waves break, exhaling as they pull back.

Concentrate on the sun as it sinks below the horizon. The yellow rays have now turned to a deep orange, shooting like blazing arrows across the darkening sky, their reflection giving a warm, fiery glow to the ocean below. On your next inhalation, visualize these orange arrows of light penetrating your Sacral chakra to cleanse and vivify it as they swirl around its centre in a clockwise movement.

Exhale, breathing out any negativity and stagnant energy that these rays have uncovered. If you know the cause of this stagnation, you need to find ways to resolve the cause. Sometimes residual energy can stem from situations in the distant past. Let the orange rays gently disperse the unwanted energy.

Bring your awareness back to the horizon as the dark indigo of night wraps you in a cloak of peace.

STIMULATING ASANAS

The yoga postures (*asanas*) shown here have been chosen as they work directly with the Sacral chakra. Physically they work with the hamstring muscles at the back of the legs. To make these muscles supple sometimes takes a lot of practice.

When working with these postures, it is important that you bend from the hips and not from the thoracic spine. Tension in the lower part of the body can make this difficult, but the position of the body before and during a posture is more important than how far you are able to extend into the posture.

When working with Padangusthasana, make sure that the weight of your body is distributed equally on the front of both feet. This will help to keep your hips in line with your ankles.

When you have extended as far into the posture as is possible for you, breathe normally and bring your concentration into your Sacral chakra. With each inhalation, visualize a ray of orange light coming through your feet and into the chakra to strengthen and vivify it. Work with this visualization for as long as you are able to maintain the posture. Then inhale and return to either a standing or sitting posture.

PADANGUSTHASANA
HAND TO FOOT POSTURE

CAUTION:
Do not practise
if you suffer
from sciatica.

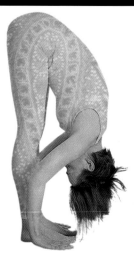

❶ *Begin in standing posture (see page 15).*

❷ *Inhale and lift up your spine then exhale, bending the trunk of your body forward from the hips, keeping your spine straight and your knees locked.*

❸ *Try to hold your big toes with your hands.*

❹ *Inhale, then on your next exhalation continue to lower the trunk of your body on to your legs, placing your hands on either side of your feet to lie flat on the ground.*

BENEFITS:

This posture eases constipation and indigestion, increases suppleness of the back muscles and stimulates the spinal nerves. It can help sexual ailments and increase blood supply to the brain.

JANU SIRASANA
HEAD TO KNEE POSTURE

PASCHIMOTTANASANA
BACK STRETCHING POSTURE

CAUTION:
Do not practise if you suffer from sciatica.

CAUTION:
Do not practise if you suffer from sciatica, a slipped disc or chronic arthritis.

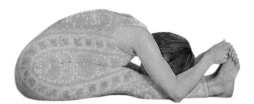

1 Sit on the floor with your legs extended in front of your body.

2 Bend your right knee and place the sole of your right foot against the thigh of your left leg with your right knee on the floor. (If you are unable to touch the floor with your right knee, support it with a cushion or blanket.)

3 Inhaling, straighten the spine and extend both hands to hold the left foot. (If you cannot reach your foot, place a belt around it and hold either end.)

4 Exhaling, and keeping your spine straight, gently lower the trunk of your body on to the left leg, keeping the knee locked.

5 On your next inhalation raise the trunk of your body back to sitting posture. Repeat on your left side by bending your left knee.

1 Sit on the floor with your legs extended in front of you.

2 Inhaling, straighten your spine and take your hands down to your feet. (If you are unable to touch your feet, work with a belt as described in the previous exercise.)

3 Keeping your spine straight and your knees locked, exhale and slowly lower the trunk of your body until it is lying flat along your legs. Hold this posture whilst working with your visualization exercise. When you are ready, inhale and come back to the sitting posture.

BENEFITS:

This posture eases constipation and indigestion, increases suppleness of the back muscles and stimulates the spinal nerves. It can help sexual ailments and increase blood supply to the brain.

BENEFITS:

This posture may help with weight loss in the abdominal region. It tones the abdominal organs, activates the kidneys, liver, pancreas and adrenal glands.

BREATH AND SOUND

Our breath is reputed to be the most important step between body and spirit. Many ancient cultures were aware of the power of the breath and utilized it to raise their level of consciousness and to heal. The ancient Greeks believed the diaphragm to be the seat of the soul, and many mystics believed that specific forms of breathing led one to experience the true self.

The way we breathe determines our mental and physical well-being. When nervous, our breathing becomes shallow and agitated, depriving us of oxygen and *prana*. Deepening our breathing, with the aid of the exercises in this book, increases the blood's oxygen levels and reduces anxiety.

Starting to work with breathing exercises may cause physical changes, increase sensitivity and make you more receptive to the energy fields surrounding you. Initially, it may be difficult to remain focused on the breath, but this will improve with practice.

The yoga complete breath (*right*) is the next step on from the rhythmic breath.

THE COMPLETE BREATH

Sitting in simple cross-legged posture (see page 14), gently release the tension from your body. Bring your concentration to your breath and take a few slow inhalations and exhalations to calm your mind and relax your body.

Breathe out fully, contracting your abdominal muscles to rid the lungs of as much air as possible. Slowly breathe in to a count of seven, allowing your abdomen to relax and swell out to make room for your descending diaphragm.

Sense your lungs filling from the very bottom to the top with air. Hold your breath in for a count of two. Exhale slowly to a count of seven, expelling the air in your lungs and finally contracting the muscles of your abdomen again to expel as much stale air as possible. Hold out for a count of two before starting your next inhalation.

When you become familiar with this technique, try to take notice of the effect that it has on your Sacral chakra and your abdominal muscles.

MANTRA EXERCISE

The mantra for the sacral chakra is Vam, although the vowel sound 'Ooo' (as in 'you') can be used as an alternative.

Sitting quietly, start with a few rounds of the yoga complete breath (left). When you are ready, inhale fully, then, on a slow exhalation, start to intone the vowel 'Ooo'. If possible intone this on D above middle C. This is one tone higher than the note used for the Base chakra.

Make your intonation soft and gentle and try to feel where in your body it is resonating. Experiment with the pitch until you feel the vibration in and around your abdomen. Now bring your concentration to your Sacral chakra and project the sound there. Sense the vibration of sound bringing this centre into balance. Initially, you should practise this technique for approximately five minutes, but this time can be extended as you become more proficient.

Now change the sound to Vam (as in 'ham'). Start with your mouth slightly open to sound the first two letters 'Va', gradually closing your mouth and bringing your lips together to sound the 'm', holding this sound for the full exhalation of your breath – Vammm. Continue with this sound for a further two to three minutes, then take note of which of these two sounds had the greatest effect.

It is advisable to work with both sounds for a few weeks, alternating them with each practice session. If you then find that one sound works better for you, concentrate on that. Each chakra is unique and therefore you need to experiment to find both the sound and the pitch that works best for you.

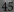

WORKING WITH THE YANTRA

The yantra for Svadhisthana is a greyish-blue circle containing the white crescent moon. Sitting comfortably in your chosen place, position the yantra diagram (*opposite*) where you can easily see it. Begin by fixing your gaze on the blue circle. The circle symbolizes protection and blue is the colour of peace and relaxation. The crescent moon represents the water element, which constitutes two-thirds of our body weight. Water is linked with the emotions, sensuality, attachments, and our reaction to both pain and pleasure.

From the solidity of the Base chakra's yantra, we now move into the expansion and motion of the Sacral chakra. This movement links to the emotions, the water element and the moon. The moon is equated with feminine energy, which is complementary to the sun's masculine energy. The phases of the moon influence a woman's menstrual cycle and govern the ebb and flow of the tides.

Centuries of religious indoctrination, coupled with the oppression of women, have caused this centre to malfunction in many women. Working on a regular basis with the exercises in this section of the book will help to release these blockages. But first you need to have established the solid foundation offered by the Base chakra, to avoid risking the loss of your sense of equilibrium.

EXERCISE

Imagine that you are sitting inside the yantra's circle, which protects you and creates a relaxed and peaceful atmosphere. Shifting your gaze towards the centre of the circle, concentrate on the crescent moon, which symbolizes water.

Water has no shape or form of its own, but will take on the shape of the container into which it is put. It is free-flowing unless obstructed. If obstructed, the build-up of pressure will eventually destroy the obstruction to allow the water to again flow freely. If we relate this to ourselves, the obstruction represents our repressed emotions and these will restrict our natural flow of energy. This leads to an accumulation of tension, which, if not dealt with, can manifest itself as a physical or nervous disease which could eventually break the physical body. One way of releasing this tension is by allowing ourselves to cry. Crying is nature's way of letting us release tension.

When water is allowed to flow freely it is in a constant state of change. Blockages in the Sacral centre are frequently caused by hanging on to old ideas, old concepts, and to conditioning *that we should have discarded long ago. The breakdown of our daily routine and the life patterns we have formed causes fear and insecurity. This fear adversely affects the adrenal glands (the endocrine glands associated with this chakra), by stimulating them into producing an excess of adrenaline which creates a state of hypertension.*

As you consider Svadhisthana yantra, take a long, hard look at yourself. Identify and consider the factors in your life that are preventing your spiritual growth. These factors may be connected to relationships, home life, career, or ideas that you have been brought up to accept but which no longer resonate to your present state of awareness. Examining and accepting your sexuality is also an important part of the process, although it may be difficult to talk about openly.

As you contemplate this yantra, look deeply into yourself to find the blockages that are inhibiting you from flowing into a new state of awareness. If there is fear in your life, you must try to face it in order to overcome it. Fear is our greatest enemy. It shrouds us in a web of darkness, preventing the light of truth and understanding from reaching our innermost selves.

When working with yourself, exercising self-honesty is crucial. Deceiving yourself into believing that you have no problems or fears is running away from life and the joy of freedom.

To end this exercise, work with the rhythmic breath for five to ten minutes, and

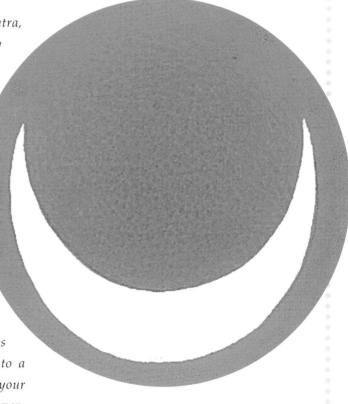

consider any issues that have been revealed and how you may work on them. Sometimes seeking the help of a therapist is of value when trying to resolve personal issues.

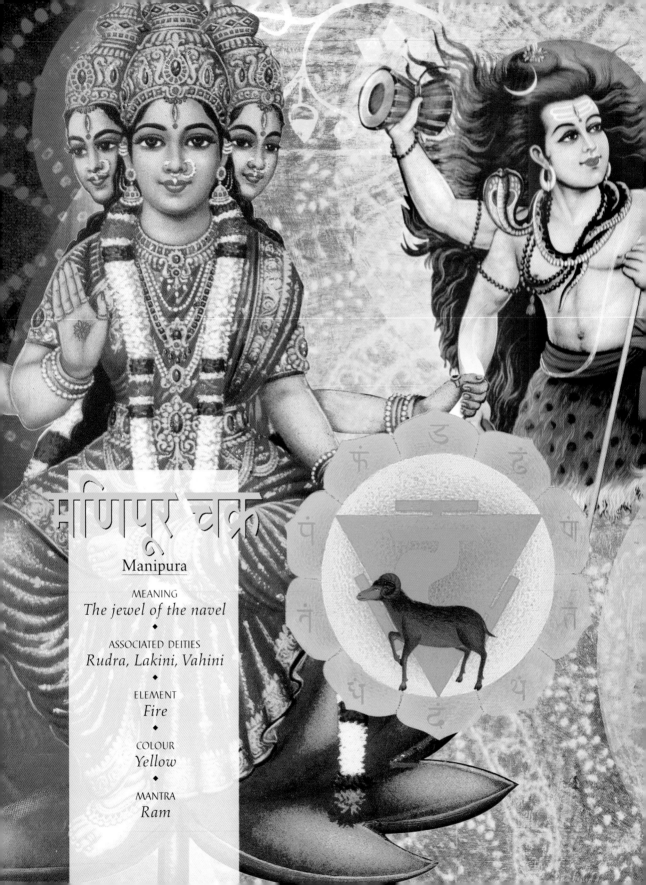

मणिपूर चक्र

Manipura

MEANING
The jewel of the navel

•

ASSOCIATED DEITIES
Rudra, Lakini, Vahini

•

ELEMENT
Fire

•

COLOUR
Yellow

•

MANTRA
Ram

CHAPTER THREE

The Solar Plexus Chakra

⊷ MANIPURA ⊶

The Sanskrit name given to this chakra is Manipura, which means 'the jewel of the navel'. It is connected to the element of fire and the sense of sight, and is ruled by the sun. This chakra is the centre of digestion, known to the Chinese as the 'triple warmer' because of the heat generated during the process of digestion. The creation of this inner flame of fire provides us with the energy needed to maintain life. When this inner flame is properly regulated through a balanced and nutritious diet, we remain healthy and maintain consistent energy levels, but if it is improperly regulated our energy becomes depleted and we can become susceptible to ill health.

Manipura chakra is linked with the ego and the emotional or astral body. It therefore reacts to thoughts concerning worry, anxiety and fear. In most people this chakra is constantly becoming imbalanced through their emotional turmoil and materialism.

Through this chakra we are able to feel the thoughts and emotions of other people, and those lacking in energy can consciously or unconsciously withdraw energy through this centre from those people they are in contact with. It is therefore vital for psychics and those involved in any aspect of healing to protect their Solar Plexus chakra.

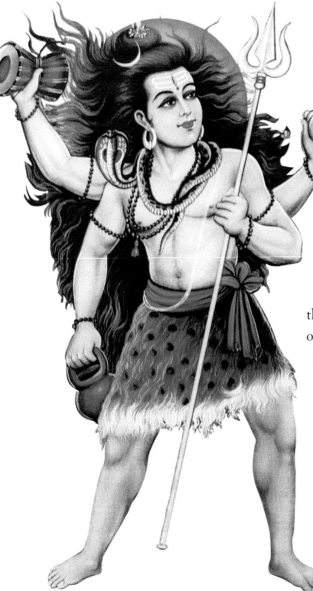

Inside the circle the red triangle with a swastika mark on each side, symbolizes the fire element. The swastika is one of the oldest and most complex of symbols. Here it represents Agni, the god of fire, and fire's association with life and movement.

Linked to the Solar Plexus chakra and, I believe, to the Sacral chakra as well, is the *Hara* (a Japanese word meaning 'belly'). It is situated three fingers'-width below the navel, close to the Sacral chakra where the fire of Agni is kindled. In oriental medicine the Hara is seen as the root and origin of *ki*, or vital energy, and of the entire meridian system, which distributes ki around the body. It is here that digestion takes place to provide the body with heat and energy. In oriental medicine the relationship between good health and a strong Hara is generally accepted.

This is our centre of power, stemming from the belief that all the major nadis originate from the navel. This is where we experience fear, making us withdraw from life. To break this cycle of fear and withdrawal, we must learn to love every aspect of ourselves. This involves forgiving yourself for past mistakes and allowing time for the things you enjoy. If you have not worked with your own passions and pleasures and are not grounded (traits of the two lower chakras), it is difficult to awaken this chakra.

This chakra is depicted as a circle with ten yellow petals inscribed with the Sanskrit letters *da, dha, na, ta, tha, da, dha, na, pa* and *pha,* representing spiritual ignorance, thirst, jealousy, treachery, shame, fear, disgust, delusion and sadness.

RUDRA

The two main deities present in Manipura chakra are Rudra and his Shakti, Lakini. Rudra (*left*) is the Vedic god of storms and has a curious mixture of terrible and beneficent qualities. He is both the prince of demons and the formidable archer whose arrows dispatched men and beasts to the spirit world. He is also the divine physician and the lord of cattle who brought the healing rain.

Many of his attributes were later given to Shiva, particularly in his form as destroyer. In this chakra, Rudra is often seen sitting on the bull Nandi, the vehicle of Shiva, but also attributed to Agni. Rudra is depicted with three eyes and his hands are forming mudras, the language of symbolic hand gestures and movements for granting boons and dispelling fear.

Rudra is often of a red hue, but here he is depicted looking old and white from the ashes that cover him. The ashes serve to remind us of our need to transform through the fire of purification any fear and egoism that we have centred here, so that our renewed energies can rise to the Heart chakra. We are also invited to contemplate the reality of death, the portal through which all of us must pass when our eternal self returns to the spiritual world and our physical body to the dust and ashes from which it was formed.

Another form of death, which we need to think about when working with this chakra, is dying to our physical self. That is, learning to put the material and physical aspects of our lives below our spiritual and emotional needs. This is important if we are to recognize our eternal self, our source of origin and the purpose for our present incarnation. This is the ultimate aim of chakra work, yoga and all the great religions of the world.

LAKINI

Sitting next to Rudra on a red lotus flower is the goddess Lakini (*see page 48, left*). She is depicted with three heads, each bearing three eyes, and four arms. Her three heads invite us to become aware of the physical, the astral and the celestial planes. In one of her hands she holds the thunderbolt, symbolic of the electrical energy of fire and the physical heat that is said to radiate from her body; another holds the *sakti*, the weapon of fire. Her other two hands form the hand movements or mudras for allaying fears and granting blessings. Traditionally believed to be fond of meat, her breast is red with the blood and fat that drops from her mouth.

VAHINI

Vahini, the nature god, is also often shown inside the triangle of Manipura chakra as shining red and riding on the back of a ram. Vahini has four arms in which he holds a rosary and a spear and shows the gesture of granting boons and dispelling fear. He is connected to the fire element and the mantra 'Ram'. The ram is connected to the sacred fire and Agni.

ENERGIZING MANIPURA

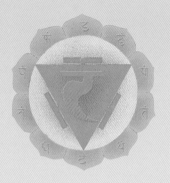

P arts of the body influenced by this chakra are the skin, digestive organs, stomach, duodenum, pancreas, liver, and the endocrine glands, the Islets of Langerhans, which are responsible for the production of insulin within the pancreas. The opposing forces of this chakra are power and weakness. The following exercises will help to familiarize you with this chakra and its energies.

❋ BALANCED ENERGY

When this chakra's energy is balanced and energized you will have self-respect and respect for others, be outgoing, cheerful, relaxed, spontaneous and uninhibited. You will also enjoy physical activity, good food and show emotional warmth.

❋ EXCESSIVE ENERGY

Excessive energy here (when the chakra spins too fast) may make you judgemental, a workaholic, a perfectionist and resentful of authority.

❋ DEFICIENT ENERGY

Deficient energy here (when the chakra spins too slowly) may leave you depressed, insecure and lacking in confidence. You may experience fear when alone and poor digestion. .

❋ PHYSICAL DISORDERS

Physical ailments which may result from imbalance in this chakra include muscular stiffness, nervous tension, stomach and digestive disorders, lower back pain, diabetes, hypoglycaemia, liver problems, low vitality and fevers.

AWAKENING MANIPURA ON THE BODY

Begin by bringing your awareness to the tip of your nose and feel the breath flowing in and out of your nostrils. This will help to quieten your mind and relax your body.

Imagine you are sitting in the countryside beneath a cloudless blue sky feeling the sun's warm rays. Let the vital light of the sun energize and nourish you.

Focusing on the Solar Plexus, contemplate the spiritual aspect of the light centred there. The sun symbolizes the supreme cosmic power in each of us, which we are trying to connect with through chakra work. Eventually we become one with that cosmic power in the state of enlightenment. Imagine a golden ball of sunlight filling your Solar Plexus and envisage its shafts of light infusing and energizing your whole body. If any part of you is in pain, allow the golden healing light to penetrate there.

To end this visualization contemplate your aim in making this spiritual journey and how you now feel.

▶ *On the physical body, this chakra is situated just above the navel at the location of the epigastric plexus.*

AWAKENING MANIPURA ON THE HANDS AND FEET

Starting with either your right foot or hand, place any finger or your thumb on the chakra point. Exerting a medium amount of pressure, slowly rotate your finger on this point, moving in a clockwise direction, for approximately thirty seconds.

Still exerting pressure, but without movement, visualize the deep yellow displayed in the outer petals of a daffodil illuminating and flowing through your finger and into the chakra point for one to two minutes. Then repeat on the other foot or hand.

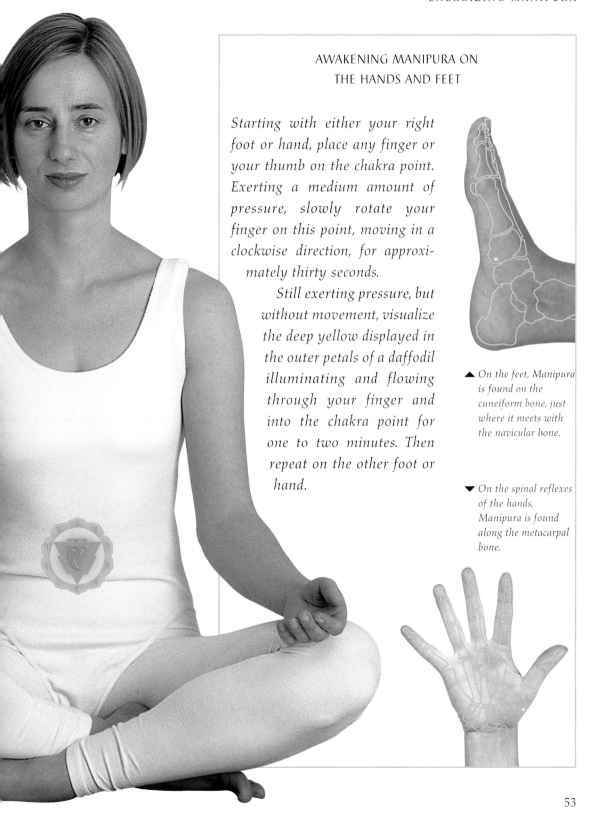

▲ On the feet, Manipura is found on the cuneiform bone, just where it meets with the navicular bone.

▼ On the spinal reflexes of the hands, Manipura is found along the metacarpal bone.

THE FIRE ELEMENT

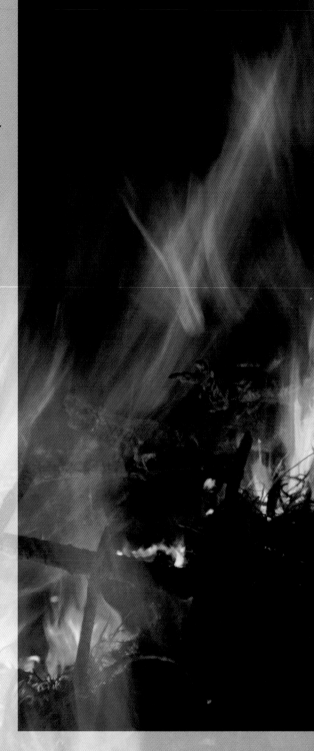

Fire gives us light, produces heat, destroys, transforms and is symbolically used in many traditions. 'Baptism by fire' is said to restore primordial purity by burning away the dross. Kindling a fire is equated with birth and resurrection, and torch-bearing at weddings and fertility rites denotes the generative power of fire.

The Buddhists look upon fire as the wisdom that burns away ignorance, and for Christians, 'tongues of fire' are the advent of the voice of God and divine revelation. In Hinduism, fire is symbolic of transcendental light and knowledge and is identified with the forces of destruction, release and re-creation wielded by the god Shiva. The ring of flame sometimes shown surrounding Shiva depicts the cosmic cycle of creation and destruction.

The Hindu god of fire, Agni, is both the rain bringing the energy of lightning and the domestic fire. The flames are represented by his golden teeth, sharp tongue and dishevelled hair and he is portrayed riding the solar ram and holding an axe, fan and bellows. The horrific aspect of fire is symbolized by Kali, who is usually shown as a fearful black or red figure with long canine teeth and tongues of flame coming from her mouth.

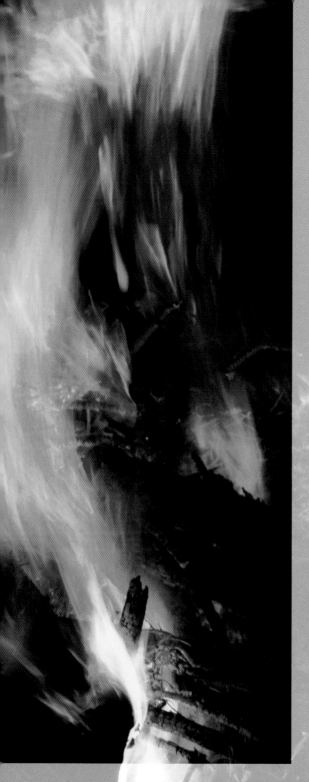

FIRE MEDITATION

Imagine yourself sitting in front of a log fire in a wood, on a clear, moonlit night. Immersed in a mantle of silence, the peace is broken only by the crackling noise of the wood as it surrenders itself to be transformed into light and heat by tongues of fire. As the fire sheds light on the surrounding trees, their ghost-like images appear, dancing and changing shape in harmony with the dancing flames.

Fire has the ability to transform and create space for new things to enter your life. To complete your spiritual journey, you must walk through your own fire of purification to allow what is cluttering your progress to be removed.

Start by examining your feelings. Where you find any negativity, hurt, pain, anger or old attachments, imagine yourself writing it down on a sheet of paper. Next, list all your negative thoughts and old thought patterns based on conditioning. Lastly, examine your physical activities, such as your job and the place where you live, and consider any changes that need to be made. When you have completed this, read your imaginary list, checking for anything you may have forgotten or are hesitant to relinquish. When you are satisfied that what you have written is a true picture of yourself, throw the paper on to the fire, to burn away all the junk cluttering your life.

If you have access to a living fire, physically write your list and watch it burn.

COLOUR AND VISUALIZATION

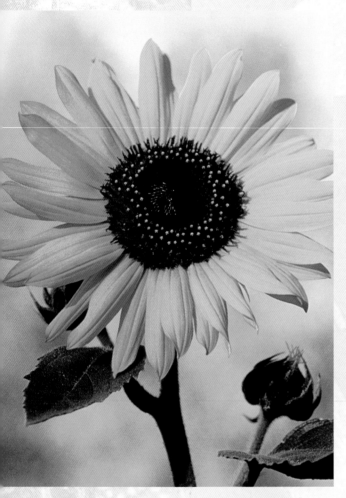

▲ *Yellow, the colour associated with the Solar Plexus chakra, can positively influence the mind and intellect. Using the beautiful image of a sunflower in bloom with the visualization (opposite), can have positive benefits for the emotions.*

Yellow is the dominant colour of the Solar Plexus chakra and is related to the mind and intellect. Yellow rays carry positive, magnetic currents that are both inspiring and stimulating.

These strengthen the nerves and stimulate higher mentality, making yellow a good colour to have in an office or study.

On a physical level, yellow can improve the texture of the skin and it can help to heal scar tissue and other skin disorders such as eczema. It is also a colour that can be used for rheumatic and arthritic conditions.

To stimulate any of the chakras' colours with food, you need to eat food of the opposite colour in the spectrum. The reason for this is that yellow food absorbs light from all colours of the spectrum except yellow, which it reflects. Therefore, to work with the yellow of the Manipura chakra, you need to eat foods with a violet skin (because these foods have *absorbed* yellow light). As a general rule, to work with the red, orange or yellow of the lower three chakras you need to eat foods with a violet, blue or indigo skin. To work with the higher three chakras you need to eat red, orange or yellow food.

VISUALIZATION WITH YELLOW

Before starting this visualization, re-read the information given on the Solar Plexus's symbolism (see page 48–51) and then contemplate the picture of the sunflower. Note the shape and colour of the flower's petals and the colour of the stamens that make up its centre.

When you are ready, close your eyes and take the image of the sunflower to your Solar Plexus. Its petals characterize the petals bordering the Solar Plexus chakra. From the brightness of the sunflower's petals, shift your gaze to the relative darkness of the stamens. This darkness creates a space for you to contemplate what the imagery of this chakra is saying to you. Think about the element of fire and the heat produced by the process of digestion and how this heat helps to maintain your body temperature. Consider the nutritional value of your diet and how you could make it more balanced.

The Solar Plexus chakra is the heart of the emotions, and to keep it in a state of balance you have to be emotionally balanced, and the master of your feelings. Your fears must be addressed and overcome if you are to proceed along your spiritual path.

As you look at the sunflower consider the other concept this chakra presents: death – of the physical body and of the ego. In many Western societies, death has been separated from life. We have a morbid fear of death and dying. In other cultures, death is a time of great rejoicing because it is believed that the soul has left the limitations of the physical body to return to the spiritual realm. Perhaps this chakra is challenging you to look at your feelings surrounding death.

Contemplating dying to self or the ego brings us to the realization that we are only a small part of the wonderful pattern of life. In realizing this, any high opinions you may have of yourself will start to fall away. In your present state of awareness you are only able to see a small part of the picture called life, but sharing your own limited knowledge with other like-minded souls will enable you, and others, to grow in awareness. How true it is that the more we learn about life, the more we realize how little we know.

When you feel ready, step back from the flower's centre into the reflected yellow light of the petals. With each inhalation, direct this clear yellow light to the chakra until it resembles a glowing ball of yellow energy.

STIMULATING ASANAS

The following yoga postures have been chosen as they work particularly on Manipura chakra. When practising these asanas, try to use the guidelines outlined below.

In Purvottanasana, aim to keep both feet flat on the floor. This is a strenuous posture and intially you may be able to hold it for just a few seconds. In Ustrasana, it is important to keep your hips in line with your knees. One way to check this is to practise facing a wall. If your body posture is correct, your thighs should touch the wall. When working with Uttana Mayurasana, make sure that your elbows are kept in line with your shoulders.

Once you are in your chosen posture, continue to breathe normally. Bring your concentration into your Solar Plexus chakra and, with each inhalation, visualize a ray of yellow light passing through your feet into this chakra to help strengthen and vivify it. Continue holding the posture with this visualization, for as long as you can without straining your body. Come out of the posture on an out-breath, then lie down on the floor and relax before starting a new posture.

PURVOTTANASANA
INTENSE BODY STRETCH

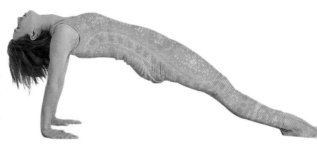

1. Sit on the floor with your legs stretched out in front of you. Place the palms of your hands on the floor by your hips, with your fingers pointing in the direction of your feet.

2. Bend your knees, placing the soles of your feet on the floor. On your next exhalation, lift your body off the floor, taking the pressure on to your hands and feet.

3. Straighten your legs and raise your buttocks as high off the floor as possible. Keep your arms straight.

4. Take your head back. Hold this posture for as long as possible whilst concentrating on your Solar Plexus chakra and the colour yellow.

BENEFITS:

This posture strengthens the wrists and ankles and works on the shoulder joints. It expands the chest and helps to relieve minor hip problems.

USTRASANA
THE CAMEL

UTTANA MAYURASANA
THE BRIDGE

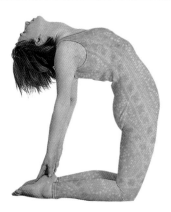

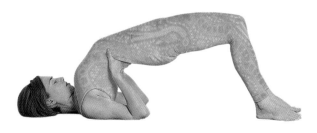

1 *Kneel on the floor with your knees and feet together.*

2 *On your next exhalation, place your right hand behind you on your right heel and your left hand behind you on your left heel.*

3 *On your next inhalation, take your head back, press your hands down on your feet and raise your spine. If you have difficulty bringing your hips in line with your knees, tuck your toes under and place a cushion between your hands and your heels. As you become more supple, you can discard the cushion and put your feet flat on the floor.*

4 *When you are ready to come out of this posture, release your hands, sit back on your legs and relax.*

1 *Lie flat on the floor, bend your knees and place the soles of your feet by your buttocks.*

2 *On your next inhalation, raise the trunk of your body off the floor, supporting your back with the palms of your hands.*

3 *Make sure that your hands and elbows are in a straight line. Keep your shoulders on the floor with your neck extended and your knees together.*

4 *Hold the posture for as long as is comfortable, concentrating on Manipura chakra and the colour yellow. If you have difficulty with this posture, place a wooden block or a thick book beneath the lower part of your lumbar spine, and place your arms by the side of your raised body. Practise with this until your arms become strong enough to support your body.*

BENEFITS:

This posture stretches and tones the whole of the spine, making it supple. It also works on the abdominal organs and muscles and on the shoulder joints.

BENEFITS:

This posture strengthens and improves flexibility in the back and wrist joints. It also tones the abdominal organs and works the thigh muscles.

BREATH AND SOUND

Before working with the yantra given on pages 62–3, it is beneficial to clear the Manipura chakra of the undesirable emotions of fear, worry, anxiety, hate, anger, jealousy, envy, melancholy, excitement and grief.

To start this process, reach into yourself to detect the presence of any of these negative emotions. Suppressing or ignoring such feelings can be detrimental to your health, especially if you have managed to bury them in your unconscious mind. Normally we suppress such feelings, either through a sense of guilt or because they are too painful to deal with. But ultimately they have to be uncovered and worked through in order to clear the chakra of stagnant energy. The following breathing exercises will help you to do this if practised regularly.

CLEARING THE SOLAR PLEXUS

Bring your concentration to your Solar Plexus and work with the Rhythmic Breath (see page 28–9) for two to three minutes.

On your next exhalation, send the mental command 'Get out!' to any negativity residing in your Solar Plexus. This command must be forceful and truly meant. Visualize any undesired emotions being carried away with the exhaled breath.

Repeat this seven to ten times before checking for any remaining, unwanted emotions. If need be, repeat the exercise. Follow this exercise with the cleansing breath described below.

THE CLEANSING BREATH

This breathing exercise will cleanse and ventilate your lungs, stimulate connected cells and generally improve the condition of the respiratory organs. It is particularly beneficial when you are tired and drained of energy.

Exhale completely to rid the lungs of carbon dioxide and other waste products. Inhale slowly and completely. Pucker up your lips without swelling out your cheeks, as if you are going to whistle, then exhale a small amount of air, with great force, through your puckered lips.

Retain the remaining air for a moment before exhaling a little more. Repeat this until all the air from your lungs is completely exhaled.

MANTRA EXERCISE

The Sanskrit mantra for Manipura chakra is 'Ram' which, when intoned, is said to vivify the sun energy of this centre. Another sound that can be intoned is 'Aw' (pronounced as in 'core'). Initially you may find it simpler to start with this sound

Sitting quietly, take a deep breath and, as you slowly exhale, start to intone the sound, Aw. On your next inhalation bring your concentration to your Solar Plexus chakra. Exhaling, repeat this sound. Experiment with different pitches until you find the sound that resonates with this chakra. When you have found the right pitch, continue to work with it for a further ten to fifteen rounds. Now change to the mantra Ram. After completing a further ten to fifteen rounds, contemplate which sound feels right for you.

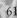

WORKING WITH THE YANTRA

The yantra for this chakra can be either the swastika or the downward-pointing triangle. The swastika is one of the oldest and most complex of symbols and is used widely by Buddhists and devotees of Vishnu. Its exact symbolism is unknown but many interpretations surround it. It appears with both gods and goddesses but is associated mainly with solar and generative symbols such as the lion, ram, deer, horse, birds and the lotus.

The swastika is said to be the cross of India, and is the sign of Pisces in the Indian zodiac. In Hinduism it is the symbol of the fire god Agni, as well as being associated with Brahma, Surya, Vishnu and Ganesh, the pathfinder and god of the crossroads.

The swastika's triangle symbolizes the law of balance and is geometrically the equal of the number three. In Christianity it represents the trinity of God the Father, God the Son and God the Holy Spirit; in Hinduism it is Brahma the creator, Vishnu the preserver and Shiva the destroyer, and in humans it is body, mind and spirit. In its three dimensional form it becomes the tetrahedron, the platonic solid symbolizing fire. The upward-facing triangle represents the sun and the masculine energy and the downward-pointing triangle the moon and feminine energy. The visualization, right, will allow you to harness the power of this chakra.

EXERCISE

Fire, the element connected with this chakra, gives us light, produces heat, transforms and is therefore essential to life. At the solar-plexus chakra it is symbolized by the triangle which points downwards.

Spiritually, there are two kinds of fire: the first is the fire of earth, the fire of our base desires which devours and reduces to ashes whatever it touches. This is sometimes referred to as the fire of passion, which can inflict great suffering if we are not prepared to relinquish our desires. The second is the celestial fire of the sun, the sacred fire of divine love which enables us to be transformed into a spritual, radiant being.

Position the yantra where you can see it comfortably, then light a candle and stand this either on a table or on the floor in front of you. As you contemplate the flame of the candle, consider the two kinds of fire mentioned above. The first, the fire of passion can be founded on materialism or it can be ignited through a great desire to discover who you really are and the true aim of your earthly life. If based on materialism and selfish desires, then these need to be transformed. This you can do by walking through the divine fire of purification, and visualizing all your negative attributes being consumed by the flames. To work successfully with the heart chakra next, you must work to transcend the three lower chakras. Part of this process is working with the transforming power of fire.

Still looking at the candle flame, think about your own inner flame of light, a reflection of your spiritual life and work. The strength of this flame reflects your spiritual growth, achieved through your many incarnations into a physical form. If the flame is strong, it will withstand the many challenges you are given, but if weak, the storms of life could extinguish it. Each time you incarnate, you are given opportunities for growth but you are also given free will to accept or reject these opportunities.

Shifting your gaze to the yantra, imagine yourself standing on the outside of the circle. Visualize the triangle surrounded with the celestial flames of purification. These brilliant, dancing yellow, red and orange flames invite you to walk through them. If you chooose to do this, their light will reveal what you need to transform in your life to raise your energies to

the heart chakra. As you acknowledge the changes that need to be made, ponder ways of doing this. This can be a very painful process, especially if the changes threaten your security, but remember, ultimately your security must come from within yourself and not from outside.

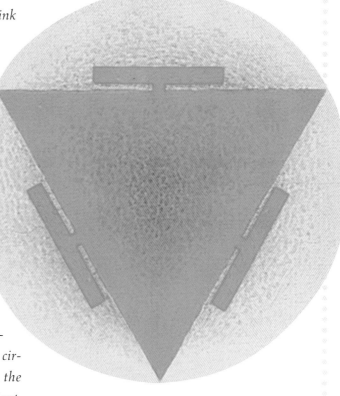

Finally, take one of these celestial flames and unite it with your own inner flame of light. Strengthen and nurture this flame with daily meditation and contemplation.

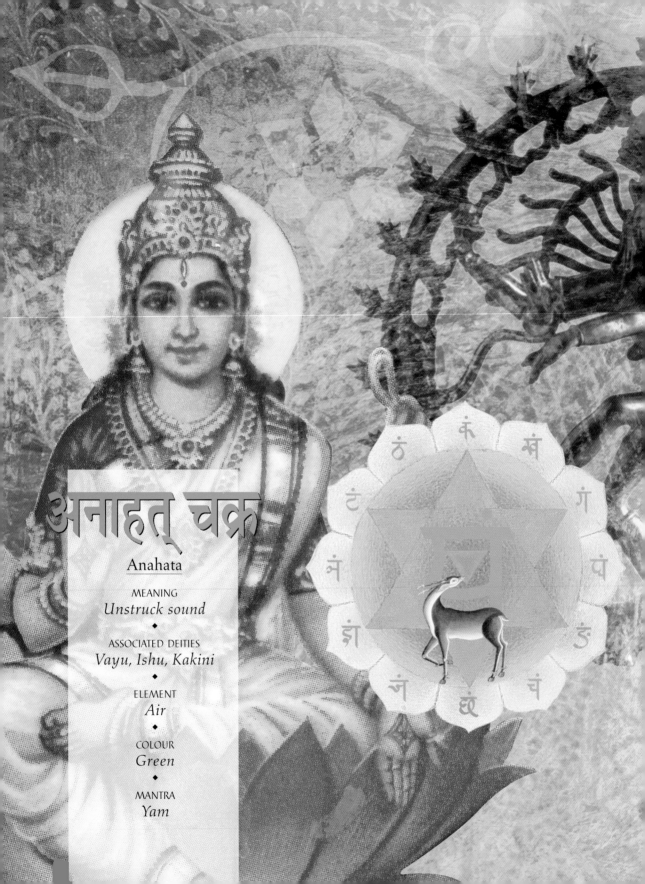

अनाहत चक्र

Anahata

MEANING
Unstruck sound

◆

ASSOCIATED DEITIES
Vayu, Ishu, Kakini

◆

ELEMENT
Air

◆

COLOUR
Green

◆

MANTRA
Yam

CHAPTER FOUR

The Heart Chakra

⇒⊶ ANAHATA ⊷⇐

The Sanskrit name for this chakra is Anahata, which means the unstruck or unbeaten sound. Sound in the universe is produced by the striking together of objects. This sets up vibrations or sound waves. But the sound that comes from beyond this material world, known as the primordial sound, is the source of all sound. It is the Anahata sound. The Heart chakra is the centre of balance and equilibrium. The three chakras below the Heart chakra are mainly concerned with instinctual nature, and the three above relate to a higher or more evolved state of consciousness.

This chakra is shown as a circle surrounded by twelve green petals, bearing in black Sanskrit letters the sounds *k, kh, g, gh, n, ch, chh, j, jh, n, t* and *th*. The twelve modes of being associated with this chakra are lustfulness, fraudulence, indecision, repentance, hope, anxiety, longing, impartiality, arrogance, incompetence, discrimination and defiance.

Inside the circle is the smoky blue hexagon constructed by interlacing the downward- and upward-pointing triangles. The downward-pointing triangle signifies the lower nature of humans and is connected to the earth energies, and the upper triangle represents the higher nature and is linked to our spiritual energies.

The interlaced triangle characterizes the union of opposites, 'as above, so below'. It stands for the perfect balance of complementary forces and the androgynous nature of the one true deity of which all the gods are incarnations. The upward-pointing triangle is solar energy and fire, and embodies the masculine principle and the downward-pointing triangle is linked with the moon, water and the feminine principle.

The second polarity in this chakra is that which exists between right and left. The right is masculine and yang in nature and the left is feminine with yin characteristics. If we were to draw a vertical line to separate our left and right sides and a horizontal line to separate the three lower and the three upper chakras, we would create a cross symbolizing all aspects of our self. It is all these aspects that become integrated at the heart centre through the power of unconditional love.

THE GOD VAYU

In some representations of this mantra, Vayu, the god of the wind and master of the mantra Yam, is shown inside the hexagon. He is a smoky colour and rides upon a black antelope. Vayu is also often shown with four arms, and carrying the goad. The antelope is noted for its fleetness and motion – attributes which link it with the air element. The black antelope is the emblem of Shiva and is purported to pull the chariots of the sun and the moon.

SHIVA AS ISHU

The other deities are Ishu and Kakini. Ishu is another form of Shiva. In his representation as Ishu he is the overlord of the three lower chakras. He is often depicted with two arms and three eyes. The third eye, situated in his forehead, is his eye of wisdom. With his hands he forms mudras, one for granting boons and the other for removing fear. In some representations he is clad in silken raiment, with bells on his toes and many jewels around his neck.

LORD OF THE DANCE

Another name by which Shiva is known is 'Lord of the Dance'. This title is relevant to this chakra because his dance symbolizes divine activity as the source of movement in the universe, particularly under the aspect of the cosmic functions of creation, conservation, destruction, incarnation and liberation. Sometimes Shiva dances where cremations take place to draw the demons and earthbound spirits – said to haunt these places – into the dance to neutralize their evil powers. He is shown in this guise on pages 64–65.

The Heart chakra can also be likened to a place of cremation where our sense of self and all the negativity that stems from this is consumed. It is also where the material aspects of the three lower chakras are transformed in the fire, to free our soul to identify itself with the divine lord of the dance. It has been said that the supreme and perfect rhythm of the dynamic and triumphant joy that follows this purification is better expressed through dance than with words.

KAKINI

The goddess Kakini *(right)*, the feminine deity, is depicted in shining yellow wearing an array of ornaments. She has three eyes, like Ishu, and four arms. In two of her hands she carries the noose and the skull and with the other two she makes the sign of blessing and the mudra that dispels fear. She is portrayed in a happy and excited mood through drinking the nectar which flows from the soma chakra. Again, both the skull and the noose symbolize our need to die to self, to ignorance and to the vanity of the world, so that we might partake in the sacred dance of life.

SHIVA AND SHIVA-LINGA

In addition to the two main deities, at the centre of the circle lies the feminine principle, the shakti, in the form of the downward-pointing red triangle. This has been likened to ten million flashes of lightning. Encapsulated within this, in shining gold and carrying the half moon on his head, is the masculine principle in the form of the Shiva-linga who is known by the name Bana. When working with this chakra, meditate upon the golden light radiating from the Shiva-linga.

ANANDA-KANDA

Just below the Anahata chakra is a smaller centre. This is depicted as a circle with eight red petals and it is known as the Ananda-kanda. Contained within its centre is the tree of life and an altar adorned with many precious jewels. Upon the altar our divine self is said to reside. It is here we contemplate our divinity and the universal flame of light. It is here that we are surrounded by unconditional love.

THE TREE OF LIFE

The tree of life signifies regeneration, the return to the primordial state of being and represents the beginning and end of a cycle. In Christianity, it is also associated with Adam and his fall from paradise. It is believed that immortality is obtained by eating the fruit from this tree.

Its presence in Ananda-Kanda chakra symbolizes the start of a new life, a new way of thinking. When this centre has awakened we have risen above our animal nature and reside in the joy of recognizing our true self.

ENERGIZING ANAHATA

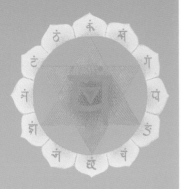

✿ BALANCED ENERGY

When this centre's energies are balanced they generate compassion, a desire to nurture others and a growth towards unconditional love. This makes us outgoing, friendly and puts us in touch with our feelings.

✿ EXCESSIVE ENERGY

Excessive energy (when the chakra spins too fast) in Anahata can make us demanding, over-critical, possessive, moody, depressed and a master of conditional love.

✿ DEFICIENT ENERGY

Deficient energy (when the chakra spins too slowly) in Anahata can create paranoia, indecisiveness, a desire to hang on to objects or people, a fear of rejection and a need for constant reassurance.

✿ PHYSICAL DISORDERS

Physical ailments associated with Anahata are high blood pressure and heart disease, lung disease and asthma.

The Heart chakra influences the lungs and respiratory system, heart and circulatory system, immune system, lymph glands and controls the thymus gland. This chakra is related to the mental layer of our aura and its polarity is incoming and outgoing thought. When we transcend this polarity, we transcend the mind and connect with divine, unconditional love. Work through the following exercises to familiarize yourself with the chakra and its energies.

AWAKENING ANAHATA ON THE BODY

Imagine yourself sitting in a forest with your back resting against a tree. Observe the tree's entwining branches, creating what appears to be an arch for a living cathedral.

The sun's rays filtering through the gaps in the foliage create patterns on the earth in many shades of green. The newly fallen leaves surrounding you display a rich green, while others show the faded green of decay. Breathe in the rich green of the leaves and, exhaling, take this colour to your Heart chakra to nourish and cleanse it. Be aware of any emotional pain being released, a sign that this chakra is being cleansed in preparation for your work with the Throat chakra. Continue to work with the visualization until you feel that your Heart chakra is cleared of past traumas.

▶ *In the physical body this chakra is situated near the fifth thoracic vertebra and is connected with the air element and the sense of touch.*

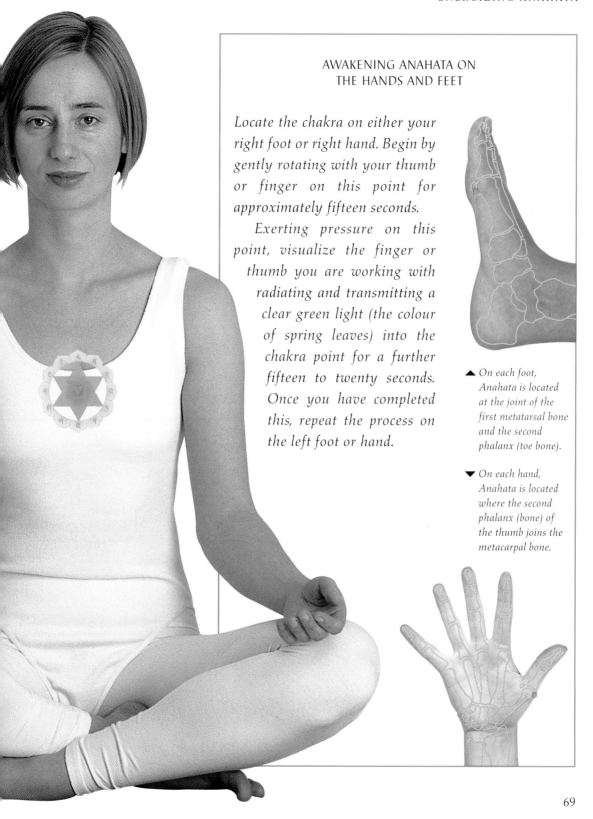

AWAKENING ANAHATA ON THE HANDS AND FEET

Locate the chakra on either your right foot or right hand. Begin by gently rotating with your thumb or finger on this point for approximately fifteen seconds.

Exerting pressure on this point, visualize the finger or thumb you are working with radiating and transmitting a clear green light (the colour of spring leaves) into the chakra point for a further fifteen to twenty seconds. Once you have completed this, repeat the process on the left foot or hand.

▲ *On each foot, Anahata is located at the joint of the first metatarsal bone and the second phalanx (toe bone).*

▼ *On each hand, Anahata is located where the second phalanx (bone) of the thumb joins the metacarpal bone.*

THE AIR ELEMENT

Air is the element that we are unable to see, unlike earth, water and fire. We can feel it but not see it. Containing the essential life force or *prana*, air is crucial to life.

Linked with the breath, lungs and heart, air penetrates the lungs when we inhale to be absorbed into the bloodstream. When the oxygen from the air comes into contact with the blood, an exchange of oxygen and waste products takes place. The oxygen is absorbed into the blood and the waste products are released with the exhaled breath. The re-oxygenated blood is then carried via the arteries to the heart, from where it is pumped around the body.

In sacred geometry, air is represented by the eight-sided octahedron. Eight is the number of regeneration, renewal, rebirth and transition. In some esoteric traditions, eight is the number of paradise. The four cardinal and four intermediate points that form the octagon are known as 'the eight winds' and the eight doors that give passage from one state to another.

The meditation opposite will connect you to the air element and allow you to feel its effect on your body and mind.

MEDITATION

*V*isualize yourself walking across a moor or plain on a blustery autumn day. Feel the wind blowing through your hair and hear how it roars across the wasteland. Looking into the distance you see a church nestling among some trees. Walking towards it, you watch the wind shift the few leaves left on the branches.

Approaching the church, you become aware of how, due to its age, it rattles and shakes in the wind. Finding the latch, you open the door and walk into the church. Closing the door shuts out the noise of the wind, leaving an atmosphere of peace.

The small church is very beautiful. The stained glass windows throw coloured reflections on to the floor and walls, giving variegated hues to the vases of flowers housed at each window. On the altar, decked in green for the season of trinity, there is a cross, flanked on either side by three white candles.

Sitting down on one of the pews you observe your surroundings and compare the silence with the roar of the wind outside. Contemplate how this might be related to your own path in life. When you are battered by the storms of life, how wonderful it is to find your own centre of rest and calm, where, at any time, you can shelter. Like the wind, this place is not visible but can only be perceived. You may return to this place when you feel battered by the trials of life.

COLOUR AND VISUALIZATION

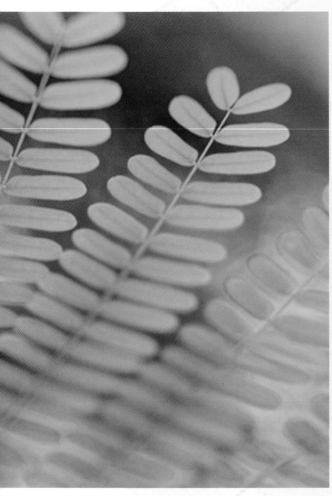

▲ *Green, the colour of the Heart chakra, is a healing, balancing colour. Working with green can help you to balance the three lower and upper chakras.*

Green is mid-way in the colour spectrum. It is the colour of balance, harmony and sympathy, and has the ability to bring negative and positive energies into balance. As the dominant colour of the Heart chakra, green works to balance the other chakras. It also balances mind, body and spirit – the three aspects of self. The greens of nature promote within us a feeling of peace and relaxation – hence the 'green room' in theatres where actors and actresses rest between performances.

The heart centre is connected to love and its colour balances our ability to give and receive love. Love encompasses a broad spectrum of emotions ranging from lust and sexual arousal at a physical level, to unconditional love that has the power to encompass everything it comes into contact with. Loving someone unconditionally is to accept them for who they are and both their good and bad traits. Unconditional love bears no judgement and lays down no conditions. If you discover that you have a tendency to judge others, then you have failed to look at yourself. Accepting your own shortcomings will help you to accept those of others.

VISUALIZATION WITH GREEN

Sitting quietly, begin this visualization with twelve rounds of the Rhythmic Breath described on page 28. This will help to quieten and focus your mind.

When you are ready, concentrate on your Heart chakra. Visualize it as a pale pink lotus flower sitting on a bed of green leaves. Walk to the centre of the flower: the pink rays emanating from the flower's petals surround you in an orb of unconditional love. Looking out from the centre of the flower, your gaze falls upon a tunnel of green light created by the light reflected by the leaves.

Leaving the centre of the flower and walking through the green tunnel of light brings you to the centre of the minor chakra that is connected to the Heart chakra, and lies just below it. This circular space radiates pale green light and contains within it the tree of life and an altar decorated with precious jewels. Upon the altar burns the flame of life.

Focus your attention on the tree of life. Note how its roots are firmly bedded in the earth and its branches lift towards the light. Learn from this the importance of integrating our earthly and spiritual lives to create a state of balance.

In discovering the joy that comes from spiritual practices, it is very easy to become so heavenly minded that we are no earthly good. Like the tree, we also need nourishment from the earth, and should keep our feet firmly planted. This tree's branches represent the many challenges that life offers, to help us evolve along our chosen path. We can reject or accept these challenges. However, rejecting challenges only delays them.

From the tree of life, shift your gaze to the altar flame. Observe how it moves and how the current of air flowing through this chakra fans the flame to glow more brightly. The strength of the flame enables it to withstand this current and grow stronger. Consider the strength of your inner flame of light. Is it strong enough to withstand the storms of life or is it so weak that it is in danger of going out?

Before ending this visualization, think about your own inner flame of light. Consider how you can work to make it brighter and stronger so that it is not in danger of being extinguished by the hardships of life. Each time you work with this exercise, imagine your inner flame growing bigger, brighter and stronger.

STIMULATING ASANAS

The following asanas work with the Heart chakra. Before attempting these postures, take note of the cautions. Work slowly and carefully with each posture. Try to keep concentrated on the posture you are working with. If your mind wanders, bring it back to the task in hand.

When working with Utthita Trikonasana, remember to rotate your body from your waist without altering the position of your hips. Make sure that your chest is facing the opposite wall, and not down towards the floor. If you are unable to touch the floor when practising the triangle posture and the revolving triangle posture, place a pile of books by your foot to place your hands on. If you have difficulty keeping your balance with either of these postures, practise against a wall.

Once you are in your chosen posture, breathe normally and visualize a ray of green light entering your Heart chakra. Note any physical sensations experienced in and around your chest.

When you have completed a posture, relax for a few moments before starting the next one.

VIRABHADRASANA
THE WARRIOR POSE

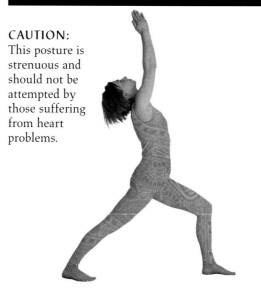

CAUTION:
This posture is strenuous and should not be attempted by those suffering from heart problems.

1 *Stand in an upright position with your feet together. Make sure that your spine is straight and your shoulders are held back and down to open your chest.*

2 *Inhale, walking your feet one metre apart.*

3 *Inhaling, turn both feet to the right. Make sure that your pelvic girdle is straight.*

4 *Bend your right knee until it forms a ninety-degree angle with your ankle. Keep the back leg straight and the knee locked.*

5 *On your next inhalation, stretch both arms over your head and join palms. Tilt your body slightly backwards from your waist, keeping a right angle with your right knee. Repeat on the other side.*

BENEFITS:
This posture helps relieve stiffness in the shoulders and back, and increases intake of air into the lungs. It also strengthens the ankles and knees and helps tone the abdomen.

UTTHITA TRIKONASANA
THE TRIANGLE POSTURE

PARIVRTTA TRIKONASANA
REVOLVING TRIANGLE POSTURE

CAUTION:
Do not practise this
posture if you suffer from
a slipped disc, sciatica or
chronic arthritis.

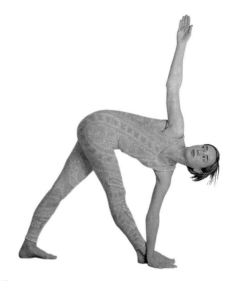

1. *Begin in standing posture (see page 15).*

2. *Inhale, walking your feet one metre apart.*

3. *Stretch your arms out to shoulder level with your palms facing down.*

4. *Turn your right foot ninety-degrees outwards, keeping your left foot to the front.*

5. *Contract your thigh muscles to lift the arches of your feet and prevent ankle strain.*

6. *Exhale, and bend your body towards your right leg, placing your right hand on the floor behind your outer heel.*

7. *Rotate the trunk of your body and look up towards your outstretched left hand. Repeat on the other side.*

1. *Begin in standing posture (see page 15).*

2. *Inhale and walk your feet approximately one metre apart.*

3. *Turn both of your feet ninety-degrees to the left so that your body is facing the left.*

4. *On your next exhalation, rotate the trunk of your body, taking your right hand over your left leg to rest on the floor outside the left foot.*

5. *Stretch your left arm up until it is in line with your right arm and your chest is fully expanded. Keep both knees locked and look up at your right hand. Repeat on the other side.*

BENEFITS:

This posture stimulates the nervous system and relieves nervous depression. It improves appetite and digestion, and massages the spinal nerves, the lower back and abdominal organs.

BENEFITS:

This posture works on the hamstring muscles and thighs. It fully expands the chest and aids balance and concentration. It massages the abdominal organs and strengthens hip muscles.

BREATH AND SOUND

The respiratory centre in the brain automatically controls the rate of breathing, so for a large part of the time we are not conscious of our breath. If we are sitting quietly reading a book or sleeping, our breathing rate slows down. If we exert our bodies through exercise our breathing rate automatically increases to supply the body with the amount of oxygen needed for the task in hand.

Our thoughts likewise influence the rhythm of the breath. Fear will cause the breath to become more rapid, but when contemplating a tranquil, country scene our breath becomes slower and shallower. Allowing your breath to find its own rhythm creates inner harmony and balance.

We all long for peace and security in our life but how this is obtained, and to what degree, is dependent upon our childhood and early teens. A secure and happy childhood gives us a strong, firm foundation for adulthood. However, we must ultimately find security and peace within ourselves.

THE NATURAL BREATH

Sit comfortably in a quiet place and relax any parts of your body that feel tense. Bring your concentration to the tip of your nose and feel the temperature of the air you inhale and exhale. It is important that you allow your breath its own rhythm and that you don't control it in any way. Be aware that the out-breath is naturally longer than the in-breath. Continue to observe this for four to five minutes.

Now bring your concentration to your Heart centre and visualize it encapsulated in a circle. The circle is a symbol of safety and security because it is perfectly round and has no corners where things can hide.

Keeping the natural rhythm of your breath, imagine you are sitting inside the circle. With each inhalation allow your Heart chakra to gently open and with each exhalation allow your breath to expand the circle, like blowing up a balloon. The larger you can make the circle, the more secure space there is in which to practise giving and receiving love.

When your circle has reached the size that is right for you, think of someone who has recently shown you love and affection. Try to recapture the feeling this gave you and then, from your opened Heart centre, return that love. When you have finished this exercise, come back to your breath and concentrate on its natural rhythm for as long as feels comfortable before visualizing your Heart chakra closing down and the circle you have created reducing to encircle your heart.

WORKING WITH THE MANTRA

The Sanskrit sound for this chakra is 'Yam' but the sound 'Ah' (as in 'car') can also be used.

Sitting quietly, focus your mind on your Heart chakra. Visualize it surrounded with the circle of protection that you created with the breathing exercise. Taking a deep breath, open your mouth wide and intone the sound 'Ah' or 'Yam'. You can use the note F above middle C or experiment with other pitches until you find the sound that resonates with this chakra. Continue to inhale deeply, and with each exhalation intone the mantra on the note that works for you.

As you intone the mantra, imagine your heart centre as a peaceful garden containing a circular pond. There on the pond, on a bed of green leaves, you can see a pale pink lotus flower. As the vibration of the sound creates ripples on the pond's surface, the lotus flower opens and gives to you the gift of unconditional, spiritual love. Continue with this visualization and the mantra before returning to the natural breath.

WORKING WITH THE YANTRA

The yantra for Anahata is constructed from two interlocking triangles in a circle. The white downward-pointing triangle is connected to the moon, water, the natural world and the feminine principle. Its horizontal line represents the element earth. The red upward-pointing triangle is associated with the sun, fire, the spirit world and the trinity of love, truth and wisdom. It symbolizes the masculine principle, with its horizontal line representing the element air.

This yantra is concerned with combining the duality of human nature. Following any spiritual path will challenge you to work with this duality. This involves, for example, accepting both your masculine and feminine energies, your good and bad points and your intellectuality and creativity.

Experiencing bad will help you understand good, sickness will mean that you know how it feels to be healthy, and hunger will make you appreciate being well fed. Life is based on experience and the ultimate challenge is to grow through your experiences so that you come closer to understanding the supreme intelligence behind all creation.

Anahata is a centre of balance, lying midway between the upper and lower chakras. Contact healers use this chakra to combine the earth energy from the lower chakras and the spiritual energy from the higher chakras before channelling them to the recipient.

EXERCISE

To work with this yantra, place the book where you can see the image comfortably. Take a few moments to relax your body and mind before this exercise.

To begin, contemplate the structure of the yantra. It is created from two interlocking triangles within a circle. These two triangles form the Star of David, a symbol sacred to Judaism, Christianity and Islam. In Hinduism it is a symbol of the joining of yoni (a symbol of the maternal womb and fertility) and linga (the masculine power of creation). It symbolizes the union of opposites.

Do you relate to this concept? Are you aware of both your feminine and masculine energies? If you have incarnated into a female body you still carry the masculine energy, and vice versa. Have you acknowledged this fact and, if so, have you worked to balance these two energies? Do you work equally with both sides of your brain? The left hemisphere is connected to your intellect and the right hemisphere to your creativity. Are both these forces evident in your life?

Consider your diet while looking at this yantra. To be balanced it should contain proportionate amounts of acidic and alkaline food, with no junk food. When working with this chakra we are reminded that earthly life must balance our spiritual life. Likewise, a life steeped in materialism prevents us from gaining spiritual insight. Anahata is also the balance between the three lower and the three upper chakras. When we work as channels for healing, the earth energies enter through our feet, and the spiritual energies through the Crown chakra and are united in the body in the Heart chakra.

Another way to contemplate this yantra is to place a symbol representing each chakra at the each of the star's six points. The three points forming the upper triangle are aligned to the throat, crown and brow chakra. The three points of the lower triangle are associated with the solar plexus, base and sacral chakras. At the centre of the star sits the heart chakra. The rays of unconditional love that that emanate from the heart chakra reaches out to the six points of the star and the chakras present at each of these points. This out pouring of love brings the chakras and all their attributes into a state of balance and will surround you with a sense of peace and well-being.

In the 'Bhagavad-Gita' Krishna tells Arjuna:

'Yoga is a harmony. Not for him who eats too much or for him who eats too little; not for him who sleeps too little or for him who sleeps too much. A harmony in eating and resting, in sleeping and keeping awake; a perfection in whatever one does. This is the yoga that gives peace from all pain.'

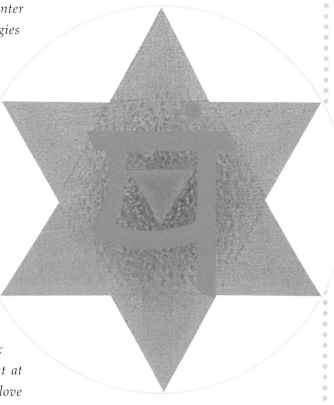

Finish this exercise with the Rhythmic Breath (see page 28), concentrating on the balance created by the equal length of your inhalation and exhalation. Sit quietly for a few moments reflecting on your yantra work.

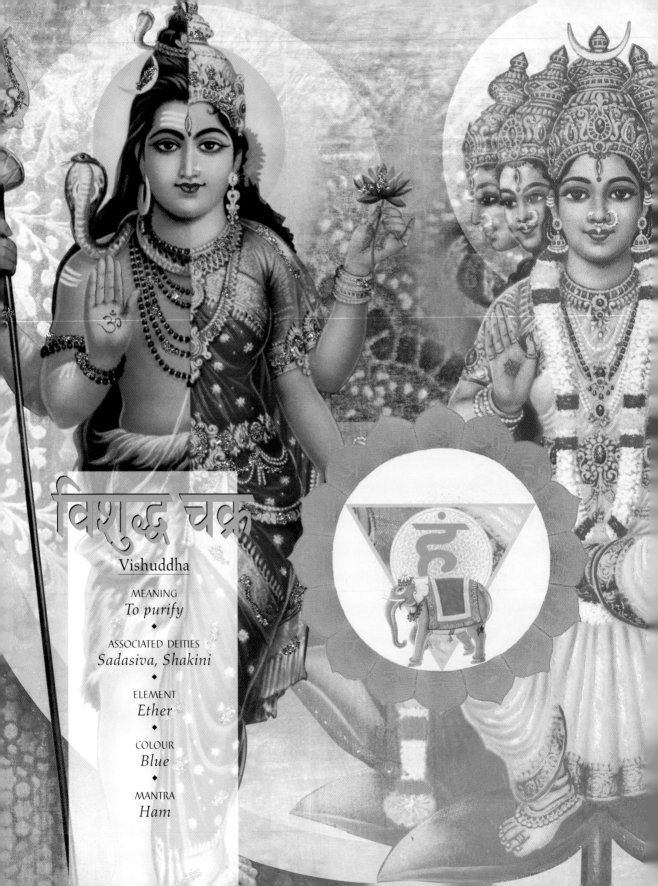

विशुद्ध चक्र

Vishuddha

MEANING
To purify

•

ASSOCIATED DEITIES
Sadasiva, Shakini

•

ELEMENT
Ether

•

COLOUR
Blue

•

MANTRA
Ham

CHAPTER FIVE

The Throat Chakra

⤞ VISHUDDHA ⤝

The Sanskrit name of this chakra is Vishuddha, meaning 'to purify'. It is located at the top of the neck at the first cervical vertebra and is connected to our sense of hearing and to the element ether, or akasha. Physically, this is the chakra that allows verbal communication but, when awakened and purified, it can also allow us to communicate telepathically and to channel information.

Vishuddha is the door or bridge that leads to higher levels of consciousness. It is here that the four lower elements are refined to their purest essence before being dissolved into the ether. The sense associated with the Throat chakra is sound, brought about through the following sequence of events. The earth element at the Base chakra is dissolved in the water element at the Sacral chakra, leaving its essence as the sense of smell. The water element is then transformed by the fire element at the Solar Plexus chakra into vapour and its essence becomes taste. When the fire element enters the Heart chakra it gives movement to the air and its essence becomes touch, and when the air unites with the ether at the throat centre it becomes pure sound.

The Throat chakra is depicted as a circle surrounded by sixteen blue petals that have inscribed on them red Sanskrit letters which make the sounds *a, a, I, I, u, u, R, R, Li, LI, e, ai, o, au, am,* and *ah* and can be intoned as mantras. Inside the outer circle is a downward-pointing triangle with a small circle inside. This small circle represents the full moon and its symbolic association with the psychic powers attributed to this chakra. It also symbolizes the element of ether. In some representations, a silver crescent moon is shown at the top of the circle. This is the symbol for pure cosmic sound (*Nada*) and the gateway to liberation.

To work with this chakra, we need to tune our consciousness into the subtle vibrational field surrounding us. Ether can be equated with this all-encompassing and unifying field of subtle vibrations. To experience these subtle sounds, find a time each day to be alone in silence. Another important aspect of the Throat centre is communication. Without this we would become isolated and lonely and our health would suffer. Communication with others should be truthful, otherwise we constrict the vital energy flow of this centre. It should also be of a positive, healing nature. A prayer influencing the chakra, that can be recited at sunrise, is the 'Gayatri', which has been used for centuries:

'We meditate on the most excellent glory of that divine sun (or source): may that inspire our understanding.'

AMBARA

The deity connected with the mantra Ham and the ether is Ambara. He is white in colour and is often shown sitting upon a white elephant. He has four arms and holds a noose and a goad to show our need to take action and to relinquish our bonds of ignorance in order to gain spiritual awareness.

SADASIVA

The diva in this chakra is Sadasiva, represented as Ardhanarishiwara (*see left*). This curious composite figure, half-man and half-woman, represents Shiva and his Shakti, or female nature, combined into one image that nevertheless represents the god alone, his essential nature being seen in the reconciliation of opposites. The Shiva aspect of his body is white and the Shakti aspect is golden. He is dressed in white raiment with a leopard skin. He is often shown with five faces, each bearing three eyes, and ten arms. He may hold a battle-axe, a sword, a thunderbolt, fire, the great snake, a bell, a goad and a noose, and he makes the gesture for dispelling fear. The lion-seat he is often shown sitting upon embodies both solar and lunar power and is placed on the bull, the vehicle of Shiva.

The presence of Sadasiva here challenges us to look at and accept both our masculine and feminine energies, an issue that has to be addressed at this stage in our spiritual journey. The great snake connected with this deity is a highly complex and universal symbol representing the integration of opposites within ourselves. The snake is symbolic of the sun and moon, life and death, light and darkness, good and evil, wisdom and blind passion and also for both spiritual and physical rebirth.

The thunderbolt and bell associated with Sadasiva represent old patterns that have to be broken down to allow for the formation of new energies. The bell also corresponds to the movement of the four lower elements in their refinement to akasha. The battle-axe shows the power gained through the transformation of our energies and the sword stands for discrimination and the spiritual decisions we need to make if we wish to continue our journey to Ajna (the Brow chakra). The Throat chakra is said to be the gateway of great liberation for one who desires the wealth of yoga and whose senses are pure and controlled.

SHAKTI SHAKINI

The presiding shakti or female aspect of this chakra is Shakini (*see pages 80–81*), who is described as light itself. She sits upon a red lotus flower and has five faces, each bearing three eyes. Robed in yellow, she has four arms and carries the noose for knowledge and intellectual power, the goad for action and control, a book for perfection and wisdom. With her fourth hand she makes the Jnana-mudra (made by touching the thumb with the first finger of the right hand and placing these two fingers over the heart).

LALANA CHAKRA

The Throat chakra has a connection with the Lalana chakra positioned at the root of the tongue and the *bindu vishargha*, a spot situated towards the back of the skull and the top of the brain. This spot is marked with a tuft of hair on a Hindu monk's otherwise bald head. The *bindu vishargha* collects the nectar secreted by the Crown chakra and passes it to the Lalana gland to be purified by the awakened Throat chakra. This secretion has a sweetish taste and the power to rejuvenate the physical body and give us full control over its metabolism.

The Lalana chakra is described as a red lotus with twelve petals and bears the qualities of faith, contentment, sense of error, self-command, anger, affection, purity, detachment, agitation and appetite. In its awakened state, this chakra is purported to have sustained Yogis who have been buried alive for days at a time.

It is written that he who has attained complete knowledge of the self becomes, by constantly concentrating his mind on the Throat chakra, a great sage, eloquent of speech and wise, who enjoys uninterrupted peace of mind.

ENERGIZING VISHUDDHA

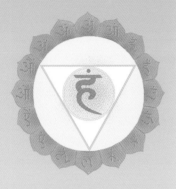

P hysically, this chakra is associated with the shoulders, throat, parathyroids and thyroid gland and is closely connected with the larynx.

Vishuddha is related to the spoken word, to creative intelligence, and registers the creative purposes of the soul, transmitted by the flow of energy from the Brow chakra. The fusion of energies from the Brow and Throat chakras leads to creative activity.

This chakra's polarity is life and death. To transcend this is to realize the immortal and spiritual self while remaining an individual, conscious being.

Work through the following exercises to familiarize yourself with the chakra and its energies.

❋ BALANCED ENERGY

If your Throat chakra is balanced you will be centred, contented and make a good speaker. You may also be musically or artistically inspired and have a leaning towards meditation and spiritual wisdom..

❋ EXCESSIVE ENERGY

Over-stimulation here can lead to arrogance, self-righteousness, a dogmatic nature and excessive talking.

❋ DEFICIENT ENERGY

A deficiency in energy here can make us scared, timid, inconsistent, unreliable, devious, manipulative and afraid of sex.

❋ PHYSICAL DISORDERS

Some of the physical symptoms that can arise when this chakra is not in balance are exhaustion, digestive and weight problems, thyroid problems, sore throats and throat infections, neck pain and pain in the back of the head.

AWAKENING VISHUDDHA ON THE BODY

Imagine yourself sitting in a bluebell wood. Observe how each tiny bell-shaped flower has an array of golden, pollen-covered stamens at its centre and is individual in both its shape and colour. Taking one of the flowers, place it over your Throat chakra and absorb the blue light from its petals. Listen to their soft sounds, observing how these interact with blue to energize this centre. If you experience tightness around the throat, it may be caused by an inability to verbally express your feelings. Removing the bluebell, contemplate what you have experienced.

▶ *On the physical body this chakra is located at the base of the neck.*

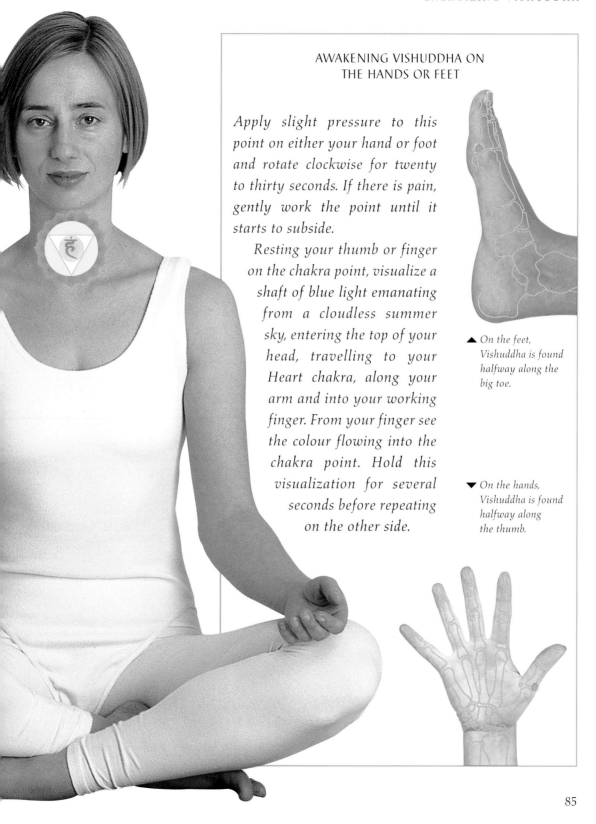

AWAKENING VISHUDDHA ON THE HANDS OR FEET

Apply slight pressure to this point on either your hand or foot and rotate clockwise for twenty to thirty seconds. If there is pain, gently work the point until it starts to subside.

Resting your thumb or finger on the chakra point, visualize a shaft of blue light emanating from a cloudless summer sky, entering the top of your head, travelling to your Heart chakra, along your arm and into your working finger. From your finger see the colour flowing into the chakra point. Hold this visualization for several seconds before repeating on the other side.

▲ *On the feet, Vishuddha is found halfway along the big toe.*

▼ *On the hands, Vishuddha is found halfway along the thumb.*

85

THE ETHER ELEMENT

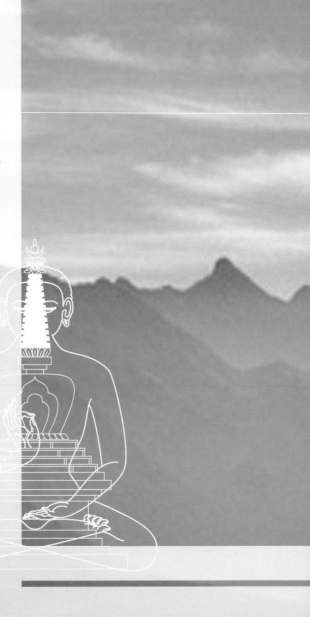

Ether is the element associated with the Throat chakra and is believed to be the element which fills all space. According to ancient Indian tradition, the universe reveals itself in two fundamental properties as motion and space. Another name for ether is *akasha*, a word that is derived from the root *kash*, meaning to radiate or shine.

The nature of akasha comprises infinite dimensions and allows all possibilities of movement. These encompass both physical and spiritual movement. Everything in existence reveals the nature of akasha and the elements of earth, water, fire and air are conceived as manifestations of this. This is symbolized in the *stupa*, a Buddhist dome-shaped memorial shrine (*see right*). Stupa means 'to worship or praise'. The shape of the stupa represents the Buddha, crowned and sitting in meditation posture on a throne.

▶ *When likening the stupa to the elements that constitute our physical body, the base of the stupa is related to the earth and equanimity; the dome to water and indestructibility; the spire to fire and compassion; the region above the spire represents air and all-accomplishing action and at the top is the akasha, the void and all-pervading awareness.*

MEDITATION ON THE STUPA

Sitting comfortably, consider the drawing of the symbolic stupa – an abstract image of the state of enlightenment attainable by all beings. Incorporating the five platonic solids with their respective colours, it, and they, are linked to the five elements of which all nature is composed.

Meditate first upon the base of the stupa and the earth element. These connect with the Base chakra, our spiritual life's foundation. Like the earth, our body contains minerals, trace elements and salts. As our spiritual awareness grows, our physical body's structure changes. Imagine it becoming crystalline and, as crystals found in the earth's darkness radiate pure, clear colours when brought into the sunlight, so the body radiates pure ethereal colours when suffused with spiritual light. Concentrating on your Base chakra, consider its colour, its element and its symbolic meaning.

Next, contemplate the water element. Essential to all life, water is linked to the Sacral chakra and emotions. Streams and oceans can flow with tranquillity or rage tempestuously, as can our emotions. Mastering emotions is difficult, but essential if we wish to flow with the life force.

Moving up, consider the fire element and the Solar Plexus chakra. The heat pro-duced from our food and the heat radiating from the sun are essential to life. The process of burning changes one substance into another. Similarly, passing through painful metaphorical fires purifies various aspects of the self.

Now contemplate the air element, associated with the Heart chakra and our thoughts. Life-sustaining air can take the form of a gentle breeze or destructive tornado. It is the same with our thoughts. Thoughts are energy forms which either remain in the surrounding atmosphere or are projected to whoever we have in mind. Positive, loving thoughts soothe like the gentle breeze. Negative, angry or malicious thoughts harm like a destructive tornado. The air element challenges us to change negative to positive thinking.

At the top of the stupa, our four lower elements are refined into the akasha, and we are travelling towards our goal – enlightenment and union with the Supreme Being. It may take many lifetimes, but returning to the Source is everyone's ultimate destiny. Dwell quietly now upon any insights this meditation has brought you.

COLOUR AND VISUALIZATION

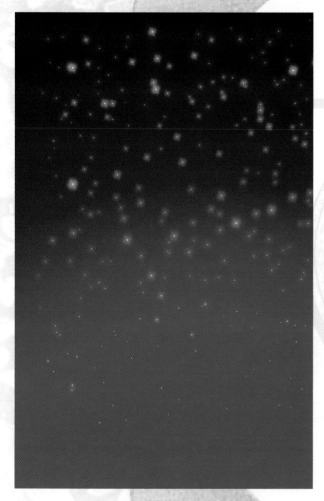

▲ Blue, the colour associated with the Throat chakra, gives us the inspiration to express ourselves fully. Visualize this colour to follow your chosen spiritual path.

Blue is the colour that promotes peace, inspiration and devotion. In all religions it is the colour given to the gods associated with the sky. Buddhists associate it with the coolness of the heavens above and the waters below. In Hinduism, Indra, the ruler of heaven and god of war, is depicted wearing a blue coat.

One of the negative attributes of this colour is profanity as in 'blue film' and 'blue language'. These sayings may have evolved from 'blue gown', the name given to prostitutes, most probably because this was the colour of the dress they were made to wear when entering a 'house of correction'.

Blue creates space and anything painted in this colour will appear larger than it is in reality, although it can appear cold. Blue has the power to promote a sense of relaxation. This makes it a good colour to use for physical, mental and emotional stress. Adversely, being in this colour for too long can aggravate a depressive state.

VISUALIZATION WITH BLUE

Ideally, this meditation should be practised outdoors, but if this is not possible, find a suitable place indoors, lie down and imagine you are gazing into the sky.

Find somewhere quiet and sheltered from the heat of the sun's rays. Lying down on the grass, look up into the vastness of the blue sky. Ponder the magnitude of space and consider whether it is infinite or if it does have a beginning and an end. Consider how little we know about the galaxies beyond our own and how microscopic we are in this huge cosmic field. We are like tiny droplets in a vast ocean but, as each droplet is an important part of the ocean, so we are unique and important in the great universal plan. Concentrate your thoughts on the sun, without looking at it directly. Consider the important role this plays in sustaining life. Without it there would be total, lifeless darkness.

Visualize a shaft of golden light emanating from the sun stretching out into the immensity of space. In your imagination, see yourself travelling along this shaft of light, out into the universe. Allow the blue light in space to surround you with a cloak of peace and protection. Looking around at the stars and planets, listen to the sound that each one makes and the gentle modulating harmonies that create their symphony. Experience these sounds resonating with the sounds made by your own physical body. Each organ, muscle and bone echoes its own frequency, its own sound.

Find the sound that resonates with your Throat chakra, feeling its vibration extending round your neck, along your shoulders and down your arms. Immersed in a sea of tranquillity, try to hear with your 'inner' ear the music of the star and planet spheres, feeling them restoring you once again to wholeness. Now bring your concentration back to blue, and think about your own spiritual path.

When you feel ready, look for the shaft of golden light and allow it to carry you gently back to Earth. Become aware of your physical body lying on the ground and be conscious of any changes to the chakra.

STIMULATING ASANAS

The following yoga postures work particularly effectively with Vishuddha chakra. When practising Supta Vajrasana, if you are unable to keep both knees on the floor, place one or two cushions beneath your head. When your thigh muscles become more supple, these can be discarded.

If you have a stiff neck, injuries to the cervical spine or have suffered whiplash, practice Halasana and Sarvangasana with two or three folded blankets. These should be placed under your shoulders and back, with the back of your head resting on the floor. In both these postures, the upper part of your arms should be in a straight line. In Sarvangasana, this arm position gives greater support to the back and helps to balance the body on the shoulders.

Sarvangasana is affectionately known as 'the mother of postures' because it brings harmony to the physical body. By obtaining a good chin-lock in this asana, the blood supply to the thyroid gland is increased, which helps to regulate it.

Once you are in your chosen posture, breathe normally and visualize a ray of blue light entering your body through the crown of your head and then travelling down to the Throat chakra.

SUPTA VAJRASANA
SLEEPING THUNDERBOLT POSE

CAUTION:
Do not practise this posture if you suffer from lower-back problems.

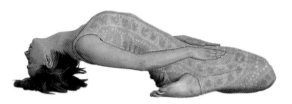

1 *Kneel on the floor with your feet stretched back and your big toes crossed. Sit back between your heels, keeping your knees together.*

2 *Bend the trunk of your body back, supporting yourself on your arms and elbows, until your head touches the floor. Do not strain the muscles and ligaments of your thighs and knees by forcing them on to the ground. If you find this uncomfortable, support your head with one or two cushions until your thigh muscles become more supple.*

3 *Arch your back and place your hands on your thighs. Keep your knees together and on the ground. Whilst holding this posture, concentrate on your Throat chakra and the colour blue.*

BENEFITS:
This is a good asana for abdominal ailments, especially constipation. It also helps to tone the spinal nerves.

HALASANA
THE PLOUGH

CAUTION:
Do not practise if you suffer
from sciatica, back problems
or high blood pressure.

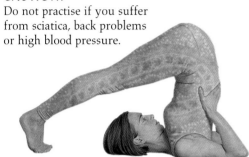

1 Lie on the floor with your arms by your side
and the palms of your hands facing down.

2 Extend your neck and tuck your chin in
towards your chest.

3 On your next inhalation, raise your straight
legs to ninety-degrees. If you find this
difficult, bend your knees to raise your legs.

4 Inhale, and on your next exhalation, take
your legs over your head until your feet,
with your toes bent under, touch the ground
behind your head.

5 Lift up your spine and support your back
with your hands. Make sure your arms are
parallel and in line with your shoulders.
Your chin should rest between your
collarbones, forming a chin lock.

4 Hold for as long as possible while
concentrating on your Throat chakra.
When you are ready, gently roll back on
to the floor and relax for a few minutes.

BENEFITS:

*This posture helps increase suppleness of the
spine and back muscles. It helps balance the
thyroid gland and metabolism. It can help tone
the liver, kidneys and pancreas.*

SARVANGASANA
THE SHOULDER BALANCE

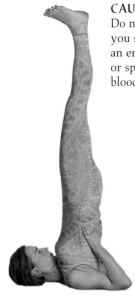

CAUTION:
Do not practise if
you suffer from
an enlarged liver
or spleen or high
blood pressure.

1 Start in Halasana, shown on the left.

2 On your next inhalation, raise your
straight legs above your head until your
body is in a straight line from your
shoulders to your toes.

3 Keeping your arms parallel and in line with
your shoulders, support your back with your
hands. Ensure that you are balanced on your
shoulders, not on your back.

4 Keep your neck extended with your chin
tucked between your collarbones to form
the chin lock. It is this that activates the
Throat chakra.

BENEFITS:

*This posture may help with bronchitis, asthma
and throat problems, headaches, catarrh,
menstrual problems, insomnia, hypertension,
urinary disorders and hernias.*

BREATH AND SOUND

One of the subtlest forms of energy is air. In hatha yoga, this is classified in five categories known as the *vayas* (winds). These are *apana vaya* which moves in the lower abdomen and controls elimination; *samana vaya*, situated between the diaphragm and navel, which aids digestion and assimilation; *prana vaya* which moves in the thorax and controls our respiration; *udana vaya* situated in the throat and responsible for expression through sound and *vyana vaya* which pervades the entire body, distributing the energy derived from your food and breath.

The humming breath, explained on the right, works with udana vaya. When practising this exercise, your concentration should be on your Throat chakra. With each repetition, the vibration felt in and around your throat centre should become stronger.

THE HUMMING BREATH

This exercise works with udana vaya. To do the exercise sit in a comfortable position such as the cross-legged pose or half-lotus posture, with your back erect. Lower your head to rest your chin in the space between your collarbones. Rest the backs of your hands on your knees. Join the tips of your index fingers to the tips of your thumbs, keeping your other fingers extended.

This position is called 'jnana mudra' and is the symbol of knowledge. Begin by exhaling as much air as possible from your lungs before taking in a deep, slow, steady breath through your nose to refill your lungs with oxygenated air.

On your next slow exhalation, make a soft humming sound like a bee. When you run out of breath, take another deep inhalation, continuing the humming sound as you exhale. It is beneficial to work with this breath for ten to fifteen minutes, although you may have to work up to this length of time. When you have finished, lie down and relax.

THE MANTRA

The throat centre is connected to creative intelligence and the spoken word. It registers the creative purposes of the soul, transmitted to it by the inflow of energy from the brow centre. The fusion of these two energies leads to creative activity. In ancient times sound was thought to be related to non-physical and physical planes of existence. The primordial sound, inaudible to the human ear, is conceived to be the origin of all matter and energy in the universe. In Hinduism, the purest form of this cosmic sound is Om, the mantra belonging to the Brow chakra.

The Throat chakra is linked with sound through music and the spoken word. Every word we utter creates a vibration in the surrounding ether. Depending on the intent behind our utterances, these vibrations can be harmful or beneficial. An example is the unpleasant atmosphere created from a heated argument or the healing atmosphere that comes from the recitation of beautiful, uplifting prose.

THE HAM MANTRA

The Sanskrit mantra for the throat chakra is Ham, but the vowel-sound 'eh' (as in 'hay') can be used. On your first practice session work with the mantra Ham, using a higher note than the one used for the Heart chakra. Experiment with this higher pitch until you find the note that resonates with your throat centre.

On finding the correct note, softly start to intone the mantra Ham. Become aware of where the sound is resonating in your body, then project the sound to your Throat chakra. Feel this centre expanding and envisage your neck and throat becoming infused and flooded with blue light.

Continue to work in this way with the exercise for a further five to ten minutes. At the end of this time be aware of the energy pulsating through and around your neck.

At your next practice session use the sound 'eh' and compare the effect these two sounds produce in order to choose the one that works best for you.

WORKING WITH THE YANTRA

This yantra comprises a downward-pointing triangle encompassing a circle and the silver crescent moon.

Vishuddha is the gateway to liberation for those who have become the master of their senses through working with the four lower chakras and their related elements. When these have been mastered, their elements will be refined and their essences immersed in the akasha at this chakra.

In the texts on laya yoga, the reverse of the above process is used to describe the process of creation. They state that in the act of creation, Shiva (the godhead), willing to become manifest in different forms, causes a vibration to begin. From this vibration comes forth the power of Shiva in the form of Shakti, his female counterpart.

The Shakti, carrying with it all aspects of Shiva, manifests these aspects with her many forms and species of life in a series of dimensions or planes. These planes are distinguished from one another primarily by the elements of which they are composed. The earth element is the densest plane and culminates in the formation of the physical universe. When we incarnate into physical form, our spirit becomes embodied in these dense states of matter in the form of the four elements. In our dense, physical body, the Shakti aspect of Shiva lies dormant in the Base chakra, symbolized as a curled serpent.

EXERCISE

Place the yantra where you can see it comfortably. Look at the shapes that it is constructed from. The three sides of the red downward-pointed triangle represent our past, present and future and our body, mind and spirit. The three sides serve to remind us of the need to integrate all these aspects to enable us to live in the now and to awaken to our eternal self. The circle inside the triangle reminds us of the presence of our dormant psychic powers which awaken when this chakra opens. All the literature on the spiritual aspects of yoga warn that these powers are a trap, and should not be desired for fear of losing sight of our ultimate aim of God consciousness. The silver crescent moon above the circle is the symbol of nada, or pure cosmic sound.

Quietly sit and reflect on this yantra and how you relate to its symbolism. Consider the three-sided triangle symbolizing our awakening to who we really are. At this time we are being called to awaken our spiritual self. I believe that the power of sound will enable us to do this. The ancient Rishis and yogis, who contacted the deeper layers of the mind through mediation, perceived the sounds of these subtle vibrations. They heard the sound of the ingoing and outgoing breath as 'hamsohamsoham' – the link between the individual consciousness and cosmic consciousness. They found that the mantra 'soham' broke through the limited, individual consciousness into the cosmic realm of Om, the mantra for the brow chakra. In the Upanishads it says that conscious repetition of 'soham' with the breath manifests an audible sound in the inner ear. Sound can create, but it can also destroy. Certain sound frequencies are known to shatter glass; ultrasound can break down kidney- and gallstones, and those who have swum with dolphins have experienced the healing effect of their high-pitched calls. When answering our awakening call, we must be prepared for great changes to occur in order that we might live in a state of self-realization.

Review your work with the four lower chakras and the effect this has had on you by way of changes that have occurred within you. Have you obtained a greater understanding of yourself and your path through life? This chakra also asks us to examine how well we communicate with other people. When we communicate, we are using sound that creates an atmosphere in our surrounding environment. The type of atmosphere

created depends on whether our communication is simply idle chatter or of a more profound nature. Do you babble on about mundane things or do you speak only when you have something important to say? When you are next with family or friends, be aware of what

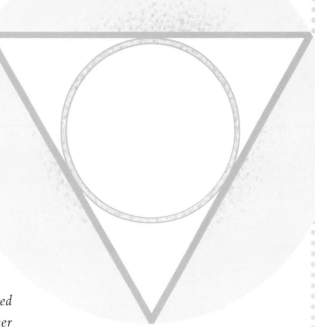

you are saying and why you are saying it.

To end your exercise session, practise the humming breath on page 92 and then sit quietly to reflect on your thoughts and feelings for a few moments.

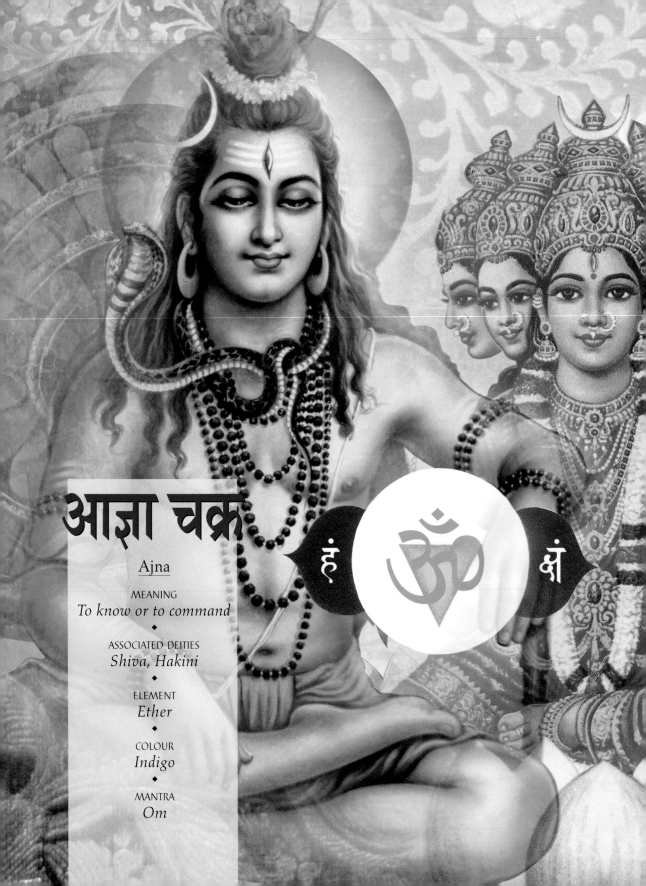

आज्ञा चक्र

Ajna

MEANING
To know or to command

•

ASSOCIATED DEITIES
Shiva, Hakini

•

ELEMENT
Ether

•

COLOUR
Indigo

•

MANTRA
Om

CHAPTER SIX

The Brow Chakra

⊷ AJNA ⊶

The Sanskrit name given to this chakra is *Ajna*, meaning 'to know' or 'to command'. From this centre intuition is transmitted to the lower chakras and to the mind. For this reason, *Ajna* is also known as the third eye, or the eye of intuition. It is the medium between our highest consciousness and the ego and between the higher brain faculties and instinctive brain functions.

This chakra is connected to the mind (*manas*) and is depicted with either two indigo or two white petals that bear the Sanskrit letters *Ha* and *Ksa*, written in white. These two petals connect with the right and left lobes of the pituitary gland and represent a conception of the combination of the two polarities of our existence. They are likewise linked to the right and left hemispheres of the brain. The right hemisphere is the seat of insight, connected with psychic power, and the left is the seat of intelligence, giving us an overview of the world. Here the celestial marriage of sun and moon, mind and body takes place, leading to the opening of the third eye and the evolved sixth sense. The three main nadis, the Ida, Pingala and Sushumna, unite here before ascending to the Crown chakra.

Great stress is laid on the importance of opening this chakra gradually. Complete mastery and balance of the lower chakras is considered a requisite. Without conscious control of the lower chakras when opening up the Ajna chakra, various kinds of disorientation can result. This book is designed to guide you in the right direction, but it would also be advisable to seek the help of an experienced teacher to use in conjunction with the knowledge you gain here in order to gain the best results.

SHIVA

At the centre of this chakra is an inverted triangle representing the fundamental triplicate of the supreme reality. These are reality (*sat*), consciousness (*chit*) and joy (*ananda*). Inside the triangle is the mantra Om. The deity present is Shiva as Itara, often shown in the form of a white lingam that resembles continuous streaks of lightning. Here *(see left)*, he is shown in a more traditional form. His appearance in some representations, at the centre of the downward-pointing triangle of the chakra, signifies the importance of integrating masculine and feminine energies at this point in our spiritual evolution.

I understand this as symbolizing the need for each of us to become complete within ourselves. When we have achieved this, we no longer need another person to complement us by providing what we still lack. If we suffer from insecurity, we instinctively pair up with someone who will provide security; if we are afraid, we look for someone to protect us from our fear and reassure us; if we are not nurtured, then we find someone to nurture us.

THE GODDESS HAKINI

The goddess Hakini (*right*) is also associated with this chakra. She is shown with six heads and six arms sitting on a white lotus flower. In four of her hands she holds a book, a skull, a small two-ended drum and a rosary. With her two remaining hands she forms the mudras (hand gestures) for dispelling fear and bestowing boons. The two-ended drum she is holding symbolizes time, sequence and the rhythm of manifest life; the skull is a reminder of the passing away of all forms of our old self and the unfolding of our divine nature; the rosary emphasizes the benefits and importance of concentration and contemplation on this centre; and the book shows the value of our memory. Hakini's mind is said to be pure and she is exalted through drinking divine nectar, or *amrita*, that flows from the soma chakra.

THE SOMA CHAKRA

The Brow chakra, like the Heart chakra, is connected to a smaller centre called the Soma chakra, meaning *amrita* or 'nectar'. It is situated just above Ajna and is depicted as a lotus with twelve petals. At the centre of this chakra lies a silver crescent moon, said to be the source of nectar which constantly flows down towards the Base chakra. It is believed that certain yogic practices enable the practitioner to stem this flow in order to gain immortality.

The deities present in the Soma chakra are Shiva in the form of Kameshvara – described as the most beautiful of all male forms – and Kameshvari, known as the most beautiful of all deities. Kameshvara is usually seen seated in full lotus posture, embracing his beloved Kameshvari. Our first contact with Kameshvari is in the Base chakra, where she resides as the dormant kundalini energy. When she is aroused, she rushes through the Sushumna nadi, awakening all the chakras she encounters on her journey to meet her lord Kameshvara (Shiva) in the soma chakra. Here they become united.

This is how the transmutation of the male seed or energy to the soma chakra, where it brings about a state of expanded consciousness, is described in tantra yoga. Traditionally, the celibacy of priests or religious leaders was maintained to transmute their sexual energies to the soma chakra and gain enlightenment.

The Soma chakra contains the A-ka-tha triangle, formed from three nadis. This is purported to contain the combined energies of the Godhead: Brahma the creator, Vishnu the preserver and Shiva the destroyer.

ENERGIZING AJNA

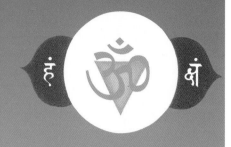

✸ BALANCED ENERGY

When this chakra is balanced and functioning to its full potential we become unattached to material possessions, have no fear of death and are not preoccupied with fame, fortune or worldly goods. Our latent psychic power opens to give us the gifts of telepathy, clairaudience, clairvoyance and access to past lives

✸ EXCESSIVE ENERGY

When this centre has excess energy (when the chakra spins too fast) we may become proud, religiously dogmatic, manipulative and an egomaniac.

✸ DEFICIENT ENERGY

Too little energy here (when the chakra spins too slowly) can make us over-sensitive to the feelings of others, non-assertive and unable to distinguish between the ego self and the higher self.

✸ PHYSICAL DISORDERS

When this chakra is not functioning properly you may experience headaches, eye problems, sinus problems, catarrh, hay fever, sleeplessness, migraine and hormonal imbalances.

This chakra is related to the brain, eyes, ears, nose, nervous system and the pituitary gland. Work through the following exercises to familiarize yourself with the chakra and its energies.

AWAKENING AJNA ON THE BODY

Sit down, relax your body and quieten your mind. Bring awareness to your Brow chakra. With each inhalation, imagine this chakra expanding until it is large enough for you to sit at its centre and become engulfed in the deep indigo light radiating from a sapphire that lies there. Let its soft, velvet colour embrace you with tranquillity.

As you look at the sapphire, you see that some parts appear brighter than other parts. Looking more closely, you find that particles of dust mar the crystal's surface. Take a clean white cloth from your pocket and cleanse the crystal. The light from the crystal is now so intense that its outline merges with its light. Sitting in this indigo light, listen to the sacred sounds emanating from Ajna chakra and feel the effect these are having on the chakra and your body.

Place the middle finger of your right hand on your Brow chakra and slowly rotate your finger on this point in a clockwise direction. Imagine that you are cleaning the chakra so that it radiates like the cleansed crystal. When you have finished, lie down and relax.

▶ *On the physical body the Brow chakra is located at the centre of the brow between the two eyebrows.*

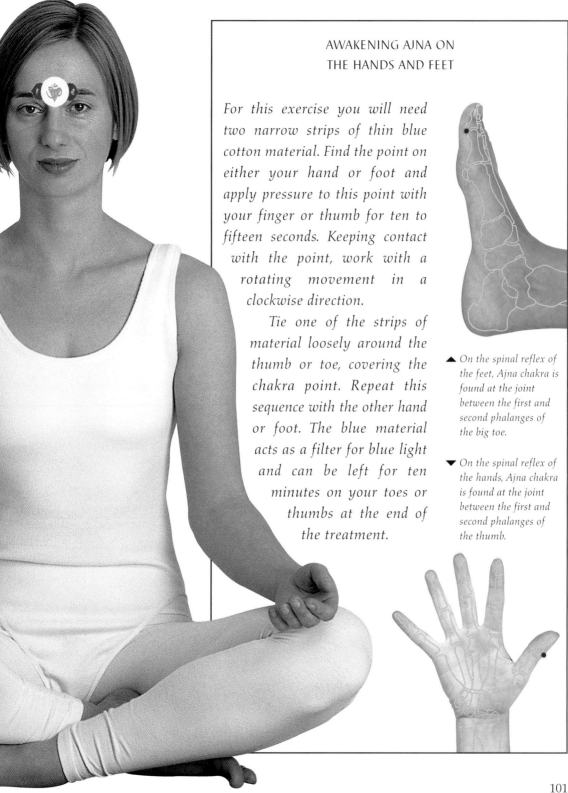

AWAKENING AJNA ON THE HANDS AND FEET

For this exercise you will need two narrow strips of thin blue cotton material. Find the point on either your hand or foot and apply pressure to this point with your finger or thumb for ten to fifteen seconds. Keeping contact with the point, work with a rotating movement in a clockwise direction.

Tie one of the strips of material loosely around the thumb or toe, covering the chakra point. Repeat this sequence with the other hand or foot. The blue material acts as a filter for blue light and can be left for ten minutes on your toes or thumbs at the end of the treatment.

▲ *On the spinal reflex of the feet, Ajna chakra is found at the joint between the first and second phalanges of the big toe.*

▼ *On the spinal reflex of the hands, Ajna chakra is found at the joint between the first and second phalanges of the thumb.*

101

COLOUR AND VISUALIZATION

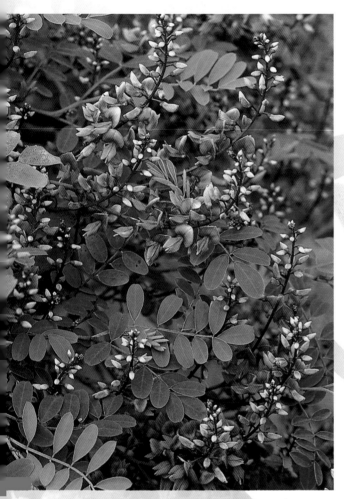

▲ *Indigo, the colour associated with the Brow chakra, is a cool tranquil colour. Visualizing this colour can develop your self awareness and inner knowledge. Shown here is the indigo plant.*

Indigo, the colour associated with Ajna chakra, is the colour of the vaults of heaven at dusk on a clear, cloudless night. In France this time was known as *l'heure bleu*, the romantic hour when ladies entertained their lovers and gentlemen called on their mistresses.

Before synthetic dyes were invented, indigo was obtained from the leaves of the indigo plant. It was a colour frequently worn by manual workers and peasants working in the field because it does not show dirt.

Indigo has the power to enfold us in a sea of silence and tranquillity and create the space needed to look at our shortcomings. Its colour speaks of deep devotion, dignity and unconditional love. It is also responsible for extraordinary vision and for giving us the ability to hear the voice of our own intuition.

Falling at the cold end of the colour spectrum, this colour is both cooling and astringent. It is a powerful painkiller and useful for easing muscular strains and tension. It is also reputed to be an aid in purifying the bloodstream and the psychic currents of the aura. It can aid insomnia and is very helpful in stopping nosebleeds.

VISUALIZATION WITH INDIGO

It is night, the last rays of the sun have sunk beneath the horizon leaving the world wrapped in the dark indigo cloak of night. The birds have returned to the trees. Heads beneath their wings, they dream of what the day has brought them. Domestic animals curl up in their baskets and kennels whilst farm animals bed down in their stalls. The owl and other nocturnal creatures are the only souls about, hunting for food and looking for sport.

The flowers have folded their petals, encasing within them the memory of the warmth and radiance of the sun. Similar to the petals of the flower, the indigo cloak of night is enfolding you within its still and tranquil energy. In this stillness, reflect upon your life, its triumphs, its mishaps, its sorrows and its joys. Take from your life's experiences its lessons and be thankful. Discard all that is no longer relevant and therefore no longer part of you.

Reflect upon your Brow chakra and its symbolism. Take from its teaching those concepts that you resonate with and leave the rest to a time when you are ready to explore further. If we plant seeds in a garden they germinate in their own time. When this time comes, we have to nurture the young seedling for it to develop into a sturdy plant. You are like a garden. Seeds of wisdom are planted in your fertile mind to germinate when you are ready to understand their wisdom. When this happens you have to assimilate and work with the new-found knowledge so that it may enhance your understanding of life and yourself.

Still wearing your indigo cloak of peace and protection, bring your awareness back to your physical body. If you are working with this visualization before going to bed, allow your indigo cloak to give you a deep and refreshing sleep, so that when you wake up in the morning your body and mind will be re-energized in readiness for the start of a new day.

If you are working with this visualization during the day, imagine your indigo cloak releasing any tension present in your physical body, relieving your mind of stress and creating an overall feeling of well-being. This will enable you to continue through the rest of the day in a state of calm and tranquillity.

STIMULATING ASANAS

The following yoga postures work primarily with Ajna chakra. Nataraja Asana and Garudasana are both balance postures and it can be helpful to work with these in stages. When you practise Nataraja Asana, concentrate on the leg movement before adding the arm position. This will help you to gain your sense of balance. With Garudasana, begin by working with the arm and leg movements separately before attempting the complete posture. To help you to maintain your balance, fix your gaze on an imaginary spot on the wall. Many people find this very helpful.

When you practise the Ardha Matsyendrasana, make sure that both your buttocks are touching the floor. It is easier to rotate the trunk of the body if one buttock is raised, but this is not correct and should really be avoided.

Once you are in the posture, breathe naturally. Visualize a ray of indigo light entering the top of your head and flowing into your Brow chakra. Attempt to hold the posture, while working with this visualization, for as long as possible.

ARDHA MATSYENDRASANA
ABDOMINAL TWIST

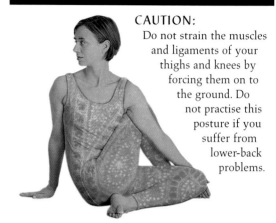

CAUTION:
Do not strain the muscles and ligaments of your thighs and knees by forcing them on to the ground. Do not practise this posture if you suffer from lower-back problems.

1 *Sit on the floor with your legs outstretched.*

2 *Bend your right knee over your left leg, placing the foot on the floor by the left knee.*

3 *Now bend your left knee and bring the heel of the foot by your right buttock.*

4 *Turn the trunk of your body to your right, placing your right arm behind your back or on the floor three inches behind you.*

5 *Take your left arm over your right leg and hold your right foot or ankle with your left hand. In this position, the right knee should be as near as possible to your left armpit.*

6 *Keeping both buttocks on the floor, exhale, rotating the trunk of your body as far to the right as possible, without strain. Look over your right shoulder.*

7 *Inhale, return to the starting position and repeat on the other side.*

BENEFITS:

This posture can help lumbago and muscular rheumatism and benefit spinal nerves. It can improve digestive ailments, and tone the kidneys, adrenal glands and pancreas.

NATARAJA ASANA
PREPARATORY POSTURE

GARUDASANA
EAGLE POSE

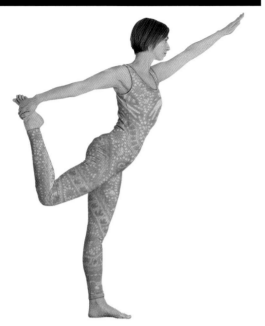

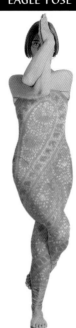

1 *Begin in standing posture (see page 15), feet slightly apart and toes in line.*

2 *Take your weight on to your left leg, then slowly extend your right leg back and take hold of the ankle.*

3 *Raise your left arm, joining your thumb and first finger.*

4 *Fix your gaze on your upstretched arm and concentrate on your Brow chakra.*

5 *Hold for as long as is comfortable, then return to standing posture and repeat on the opposite side.*

1 *Start with standing posture. Raise your right leg and twist it around your slightly bent left leg until your right thigh and foot rest on the calf of your left leg.*

2 *Now fold your arms, twisting your right arm around your left arm until you can place the palms of both hands together.*

3 *When you are ready, come back to standing posture and repeat on the opposite side.*

BENEFITS:

This posture works with the nervous system, aids balance and mental concentration and makes the legs supple.

BENEFITS:

This posture strengthens the muscles, tones the nervous system and loosens the leg joints. It helps to relieve sciatica and rheumatism in the legs and arms and develops a sense of balance.

BREATH AND SOUND

The ancient science of pranic body rhythms, which shows how the movement of prana can be controlled by manipulation of the breath, is called swara yoga. Swara means 'the sound of the breath' and yoga means 'union'. Thus swara yoga enables the state of union with the self to be reached by means of the breath. Through this practice, you can become aware of the breath as the medium of the cosmic life force. Swara yoga should not be confused with pranayama, which involves a different aspect of the breath. Although both deal with prana, swara yoga is a more extensive and precise science that emphasizes the analysis of the breath and the significance of different pranic rhythms, whereas pranayama involves techniques to redirect, store and control prana.

In the tantric tradition it is believed that Shiva first expounded the knowledge of swara to his disciple Parvati. The outcome of their dialogue produced the text *Shiva Swarodaya*. In its opening pages, Shiva implores Parvati to make sure that this science is kept sacred in order for it to remain the highest of all forms of knowledge.

PRANA AND SWARA

This is usually taught by one who is proficient in its art, and this book can only serve as an introduction to the subject. To apply this science correctly, the many different aspects of swara yoga need to be understood. Seek out a yoga class in your area to find a personal guide. Some of these cover the movement of prana in the body and its relationship with the mind. Prana manifests in many different forms and affects our bodily systems in different ways. It is also necessary to become familiar with the many techniques for controlling the swara so that the left nostril is dominant for the movement of prana during certain periods of the day, and the right nostril during the night, to create the type of energy required for a good night's sleep. Swara yoga can also tell you which nostril needs to be activated for a variety of activities and bodily functions.

If you take time to observe your breath and the way in which air flows in and out of your nostrils, you will become aware that most of the time respiration takes place through only one nostril. You may think that you are breathing through both nostrils at the same time, but this is not so. If you concentrate on your breath, you will discover that, as a rule, one nostril remains open for a certain length of time and we breathe through that side only. After about an hour this nostril closes and the other one opens. This rhythm is said to regulate all the psychological and physiological processes of the body, and any irregularity in this time sequence is an indication that a part of the body is not functioning well.

THE THREE SWARAS

In swara yoga there are three swaras. One which flows through the left nostril to connect with the mind (chitta), one through the right nostril controlling physical actions (prana) and a third which flows through both nostrils together and works with the spirit (atma). These three swaras influence us by stimulating different energy centres and aspects of the nervous system. In the nostrils three different flows of energy are created – Ida, Pingala and Sushumna (*see page 10*). When your left nostril is open you connect with Ida and your mental energy is predominant while your physical energy is weak. When your right nostril is open you work with Pingala: your physical energy becomes strong and your mental energy weak. When both nostrils open together, Sushumna is stimulated and your spiritual energy is in power.

The purpose of every yogic and tantric system is to channel the high-powered spiritual force of kundalini through the Sushumna. When both nostrils are active, it is an indication that the Sushumna is open. This allows our mental and physical energy patterns to become even and rhythmic, our thoughts to become stilled and our mind calmed. To the yogi, this is the most significant type of swara because it aids in the practice of meditation. Therefore the aim is to develop this swara by reducing the activities of the alternating breath.

In swara yoga, the Ajna chakra is of great importance because, from Ajna, intuition is transmitted to the lower centres of the mind. This is also the centre where the Ida and Pingala terminate and join with the Sushumna. It is therefore believed that our duality ceases here.

From this we can see that breathing is more than a simple physical action. For the spiritual aspirant, the breath provides a vehicle to reach the ultimate goal of enlightenment. Ordinary breathing is a mechanical function performed by the physical body, but in swara yoga the breath is a process which can be manipulated and controlled to optimize bodily health and to reach our ultimate goal of samadhi, or God consciousness.

The practice of the breathing technique Nadi Sodhana or 'alternate nostril breathing' is considered essential for swara yoga and for activating the Ajna chakra, because it establishes consistency in the breath and activates the Ida, Pingala and Sushumna nadis which terminate here. In all breathing exercises, the breath must become subtle with a slow, smooth inhalation and exhalation.

THE SOUND OF THE BREATH

The sound we perceive with our ears is only one level of perception. Many other animals can perceive frequencies inaudible to us but, they still exist. In the same way, our breath creates subtle sound waves in the deeper realms of our consciousness, which we do not hear. As the breath becomes finer, the sound frequencies become more intense and subtle and are heard internally from the subconscious realm, then the unconscious, and finally the superconscious, where the sound becomes transcendental.

NADI SODHANA PRANAYAMA

This exercise works with the three swaras and cleanses and generates prana through the Ida and Pingala in preparation for the opening of the Sushumna.

Sit comfortably with your spine erect, and start this exercise by exhaling fully to rid your lungs of stale air.

Using your right hand, place your thumb against your right nostril; your second and third fingers on your brow chakra and your fourth and fifth fingers against your left nostril.

Closing your left nostril with your fourth and fifth fingers, inhale deeply and slowly through your right nostril.

Close your right nostril with your thumb, open your left nostril by releasing the pressure exerted by your fourth and fifth fingers and exhale slowly and smoothly through your left nostril.

Keeping your right nostril closed, inhale slowly, deeply and smoothly through your left nostril.

Close your left nostril with your fourth and fifth finger, release the pressure exerted on your right nostril and exhale slowly and deeply through your right nostril.

This constitutes one round. The second round starts by inhaling through your right nostril again.

Initially complete eight to ten rounds, gradually increasing this number with practice.

MANTRA EXERCISE

*T*he mantra 'Om' is the principal mantra of all Hindu religious works and is composed of three sounds produced by the letters 'Aum'. The sound 'a' (as in 'are') represents creation, 'u' (as in 'go') stands for preservation and 'm' (as in 'mmm') is the sound of dissolution.

'Om' is the sound purported to be heard in the most profound silence. It has been likened to a pure radiant flame that turns into the white light of consciousness when practised regularly.

Sitting comfortably, inhale to a count of seven. In a steady, controlled voice start to intone the sound 'a' (as in 'are') from the back of your mouth for a count of four. Without interruption, continue with the sound 'u' (as in 'go') for a further count of four, moving the sound to the front of your mouth to give it a slightly nasal quality.

Continue by pressing your lips together to produce the humming sound 'Mmm' for a count of eight. This sound should strongly resonate throughout your head and chest. Keeping your lips together inhale deeply and repeat the mantra.

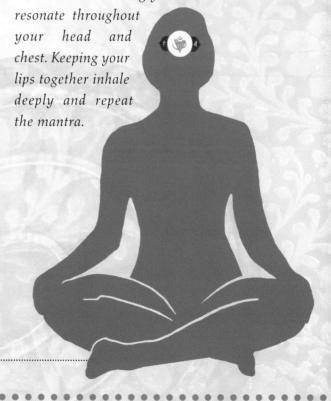

WORKING WITH THE YANTRA

The yantra for the Ajna chakra, the seat of spiritual knowledge, is the circle encompassing the mantra Om.

Your journey so far has given you an understanding of the four lower chakras and brought you through Vishuddha, the bridge to the Ajna chakra, the point where you merge your illusionary self with the ocean of universal mind to discover who you truly are, and to experience the profound peace and joy this knowledge brings. You may have already seen glimpses of this supreme state through meditation. These fleeting insights will serve to encourage the continuation of your journey of self-exploration.

On this journey you will encounter many challenges and changes, which can be painful and incite feelings of insecurity. When walking through these challenging times, the question you have to ask yourself is, who is being hurt and who is feeling insecure? The answer is your ego and emotional self. Your true spiritual self is never hurt and never feels lonely or threatened, and will press forward at all costs to your ego to complete the task it incarnated for. The purpose for your incarnation into human form is for your soul to experience its supremacy, power and all-knowingness, and the challenges you face help your soul to come closer to its fusion with its true source.

EXERCISE

Within each of us there lie dormant great mental and physical forces. Working with yoga and the chakras awakens these forces and expands our consciousness. This expansion leads to increased perception and awareness of the true nature of the universe, leading to the understanding that we are spiritual beings, forming part of the universal mind. Having realized this, we are able to merge with the ocean of universal consciousness and are freed from the world of the ordinary mind and the ego. For those of us who believe in reincarnation, we then no longer need to reincarnate into a human body, unless we so choose in order to help other searching souls.

Sitting quietly and comfortably, contemplate this yantra and the symbol for the mantra Om. Think about the embodiment of the trinity that comprises the creator, preserver and destroyer within this sound. If you follow the Christian religion, contemplate with this sound, the trinity of Father, Son and Holy Spirit. As a human being, your body was created by your parents. This is preserved during life and destroyed at death. Are you just this physical body or is it a vehicle for something greater? If you are not the physical body, but the inhabitant of it, then who are you? The first question yoga students are required to ask themselves is 'Who am I?'

In contemplating this question think around the idea of God, who was present at the beginning of time, and who needed to experience supremacy. To do this, God – that Supreme Intelligence – sent forth a vibration to manifest the various aspects of itself through the many different forms of creation. One of these forms was humankind. When it had incarnated into our human form, it made us forget who we really are. It also gave us the freedom of choice to remember our divinity through studying and experience.

In giving us free will we are able to appreciate the good by also experiencing the bad; we are able to understand joy through our encounter with sorrow and to comprehend light from knowing the darkness. Acknowledging and understanding the purpose behind our duality gives us the key that opens the way to ultimately recognizing ourselves as being a part of that Supreme Being – God. This then gives us the answer to the question 'Who am I?' which is, 'I am that I am'.

In the stillness that you have created around yourself and the space in which you are working, now is the time to ask yourself the question 'Who am I'? This is a very profound question and when the answer does come, it will be from a deep realization within

yourself. And you may not even be able to find words to explain this answer. As you take a few moments to contemplate this question, finish this exercise by silently repeating to yourself the mantra Om.

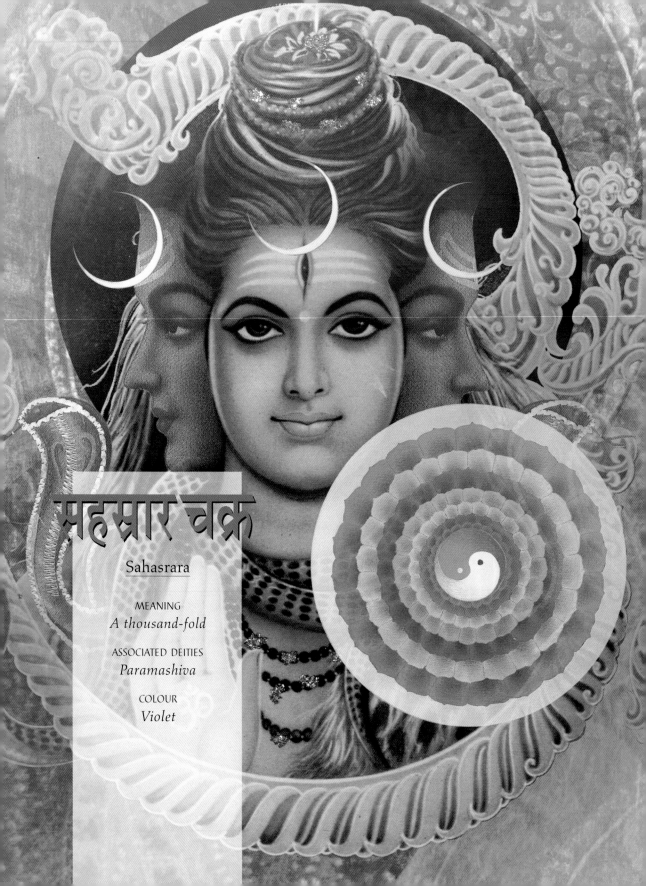

सहस्रार चक्र

Sahasrara

MEANING
A thousand-fold

ASSOCIATED DEITIES
Paramashiva

COLOUR
Violet

CHAPTER SEVEN

The Crown Chakra

⇌ SAHASRARA ⇌

Sahasrara, meaning 'a thousandfold', is different from the other chakras in constitution and effect. When the kundalini reaches this level it no longer belongs to the realm of the animal or human awareness, it is purely divine. It is the thousand-petalled lotus leading into the eternal, infinite, supreme existence. It is the seat of pure consciousness. When the kundalini rises from the Base chakra to Sahasrara, energy and consciousness unite and illumination dawns. Then, under the influence of the Ajna chakra, the force created from the uniting of these two is redirected down through the Sushumna to enable us to experience heaven on earth. Thus the quest of the yogi is attained and the meaning of yoga fulfilled.

The seventh chakra lies at the end of the Sushumna nadi and is depicted as a thousand-petalled white or pale violet lotus with its head turned downwards. Its petals are arranged in twenty rows and each row of fifty petals contains the fifty letters of the Sanskrit alphabet written in white. Inside the petals are the circle, the mandala for the full moon and the mandala for the sun. The combination of these two mandalas signifies the union of the Pingala nadi (sun, heat and masculine energy) and the Ida nadi (moon, cold and feminine energy) with the Sushumna, symbolizing the integration of our dual nature to wholeness.

Inside the mandala of the moon is the lightning-like

triangle encompassing the subtle bindu, the void. This is described as resembling a ten-millionth part of the end of a hair and is only obtainable after many years of devotion along one's spiritual path. Present at this chakra is the diva Parama-shiva, representing the union of the Shakti and Shiva.

RAISING KUNDALINI

The symbolism of this chakra is complex and has received many interpretations, all of which point to the attainment of self-realization through devotion to work and study. The symbolism involves the integrated state of our dual nature and the altered state of consciousness brought by raising the latent power residing in the Base chakra. It is important to exercise great caution when working with this energy and it is advisable to work with a teacher before doing so. If kundalini is raised prematurely, before you are ready, both physical and psychological damage can occur.

One of the great authorities on kundalini yoga was Gopi Krishna, author of several books on yoga. He inadvertently raised his kundalini and as a consequence suffered great pain for many years. It is therefore wise to seek the guidance of a teacher who has the wisdom to work with this latent power and to know when you are ready to work with it. Yogananda, author of *Autobiography of a Yogi*, mentions in his book that a request to his teacher to raise his kundalini was refused. Several years later,

when this latent energy was released, Yogananda said that if this had happened when he initially asked, he would not have known how to deal with the dramatic changes it made in his life. I believe that if we work with the right intention, the right person will enter our lives to take us on this last part of our journey. This book is designed to guide you in that direction.

To fully understand the complex symbolism of Sahasrara requires personal experience of the void present here. Mystics and seers of all religions who have experienced the transcendental states of consciousness have found this very difficult to describe comprehensibly. They have frequently resorted to using parables and imagery in their efforts to explain the inexplicable – imagine how difficult it would be to explain the taste of an orange to someone who had never eaten one.

REACHING ENLIGHTENMENT

When we finally open this chakra and reach the state of enlightenment, we are freed from the wheel of life – or the wheel of rebirth – because, having recognized our divine self, there is no longer any reason to reincarnate. Those with an insatiable desire to have access to the higher planes of consciousness will only achieve this by intense meditation and austerity. The transporting effect of meditation on divine objects, on crystals, colour, by prayer and the profound utterances of sages and seers lies in their appeal to the evolu-

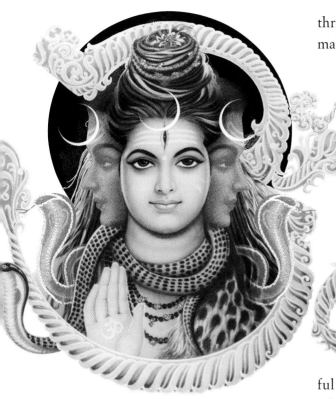

through both the right and left nostrils (normally only one nostril is dominant; the changeover is approximately every two to four hours). When both nostrils are open both the Ida and Pingala nadi are open and this clears the Sushumna, to allow the energy from the Base chakra to rise to the Crown chakra. Ideally, we should meditate for one hour. In one of his books, Yogananda points out that we have twenty-four hours in each day, therefore it should be no hardship to devote one hour to god. One learns through meditation to contact Divine Bliss by the faithful application of spiritual law. In the *Dhammapada* (a collection of 423 aphorisms), it is written:

tionary instinct which is drawing humans towards a higher dimension of consciousness, where all aspirations and ideals will find ultimate fulfilment.

It is difficult with our physical mind to comprehend this supreme state of consciousness. The nearest we can come to understanding it is through the ecstasy we are allowed to experience when meditating. We also we have to let go of this. To try and recapture the experience prevents us from reaching deeper into that ecstatic state.

The ideal time for meditation is just prior to sunrise. It is at this time that we breathe

'The traveller has reached the end of his journey. In the freedom of the infinite he is free from all sorrows, like fetters that bound him are thrown away, and the burning fever of life is no more. He is calm like the earth that endures; he is steady like a column that is firm; he is pure like a lake that is clear; he is free from Samsara, the ever-returning life-in-death. In the light of his vision he has found his freedom; his thoughts are peace, his words are peace and his work is peace.'

ENERGIZING SAHASRARA

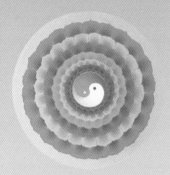

❀ BALANCED ENERGY

When this chakra's energy is balanced we become open to divine energy and have total access to the unconscious and subconscious mind.

❀ EXCESSIVE ENERGY

Excessive energy here (when the chakra spins too fast) can cause frustration and frequent migraines.

❀ DEFICIENT ENERGY

Deficient energy here (when the chakra spins too slowly) here can cause indecision and a lack of that physical spark of joy.

❀ PHYSICAL DISORDERS

Possible ailments arising from imbalance here include brain disease, migraines, disorders of the endocrine system and psychological problems.

This chakra governs the nervous system and the brain and is linked with the pineal gland, which regulates the body's internal clock. This gland was considered by the philosopher Descartes to be the link between body and soul.

When the Crown chakra starts to open, we become drawn to mystical or occult teachings. Spirituality is defined through unique individual experience, an inner knowing as opposed to external dogma or conventional religion. At this stage in your development, you may start to see auras, to experience a sense of awe and wonder at the beauty and vastness of creation. You may also acquire an inner understanding of universal truths. When fully opened, this chakra unites with the Brow chakra to form the halo often shown in religious art around the head of saints and enlightened beings.

When this centre is blocked, your creativity will be blocked and you will have no sense of your own spirituality. As a result, you may veer towards being very materialistic with little interest in anything other than the mundane.

AWAKENING SAHASRARA ON THE BODY
A simple way of working with this chakra is to visualize a shaft of white light entering the chakra and then flowing, like liquid light, down into every cell of your body.

▶ *On the physical body, Sahasrara is situated just above the crown of the head.*

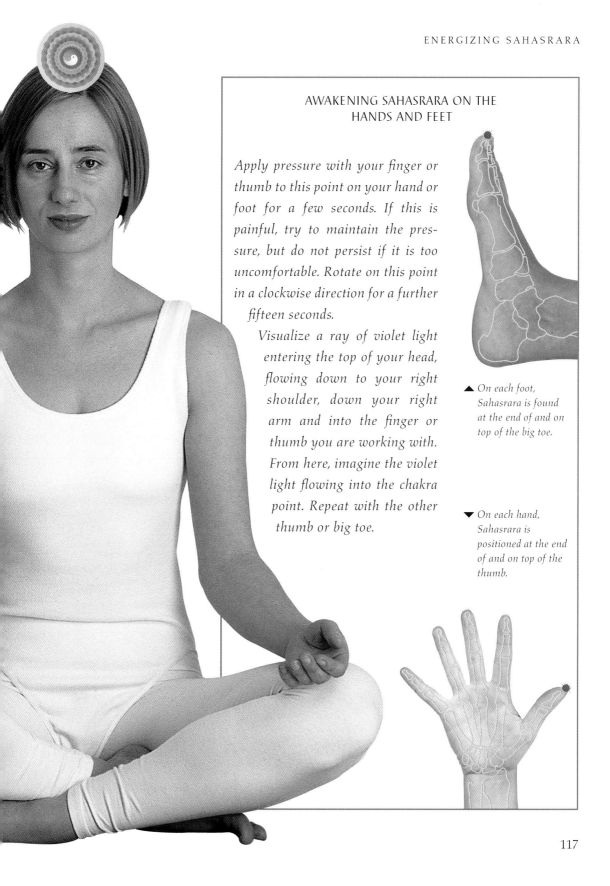

AWAKENING SAHASRARA ON THE HANDS AND FEET

Apply pressure with your finger or thumb to this point on your hand or foot for a few seconds. If this is painful, try to maintain the pressure, but do not persist if it is too uncomfortable. Rotate on this point in a clockwise direction for a further fifteen seconds.

Visualize a ray of violet light entering the top of your head, flowing down to your right shoulder, down your right arm and into the finger or thumb you are working with. From here, imagine the violet light flowing into the chakra point. Repeat with the other thumb or big toe.

▲ *On each foot, Sahasrara is found at the end of and on top of the big toe.*

▼ *On each hand, Sahasrara is positioned at the end of and on top of the thumb.*

COLOUR AND VISUALIZATION

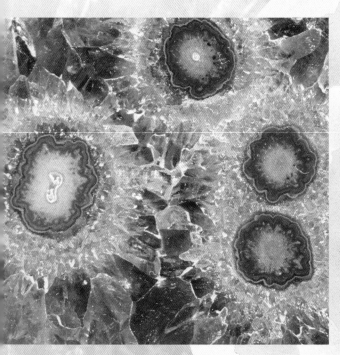

▲ *Violet is the colour associated with the Crown chakra, and has the ability to enhance a person's spirituality. Visualizing this colour with amethyst can help us to love and respect ourselves and give us the inspiration to pursue our spiritual path.*

Violet is the colour associated with the Crown chakra. The colours of violet and purple are both obtained by mixing together red and blue, and as a result these two colours are frequently confused with each other. Violet generally contains a greater proportion of blue than red.

Violet has the shortest wavelength and the highest energy of all the spectral colours and occurs in a very narrow band next to ultraviolet light. In the plant kingdom, violet is found in the violet flower, whose oil is still used to flavour drinks and candy and as a perfume. In medieval times this oil was used as a sleeping draught, and manganese oxide was the pigment used to make violet stained glass. As a dye it was very expensive to produce, which meant that only royalty and the very wealthy could afford to buy it.

This colour is connected with divinity, humility and religious devotion. It is also associated with modesty, hidden virtue and beauty. At the Crown chakra, shining violet can lift the prepared human being into the realm of spiritual awareness where it becomes the last gateway through which we must pass in order to become united with our inner divine being.

VISUALIZATION WITH VIOLET

For this visualization you will need either a piece of amethyst or to place the picture of the amethyst shown opposite where you can comfortably see it.

The word 'amethyst' comes from the Greek word 'amethustos' meaning 'without drunkenness', as it was commonly believed that the stone could prevent intoxication. This powerful healing stone comes in both light and dark shades of violet. The lighter shades can be used for mysticism and spiritual inspiration, whereas the darker shades work with the kundalini energy and act as powerful transformers of energy. The amethyst is a stone of inspiration and humility, reflecting the love of God.

Sitting quietly, either look at a piece of amethyst or at the amethyst picture opposite. Observe the shape and variegated patterns of colour inside the crystal. These make it unique. In contemplating this stone, consider its qualities of inspiration, humility and unconditional love. When you began your spiritual journey, perhaps your inspiration came from a friend, from reading a book or from your own inner need for self-discovery. So far you have faced challenges that have developed your inner strength, self-confidence and ability to stand alone. Alongside these strengths you have had to look at your humility as a prerequisite to the state of unconditional love.

Pondering these thoughts, reflect on where you stand on your spiritual path and what you need to perfect to enable you to stand free and become whole. Knowing that others have reached this supreme goal should give you the strength to walk forward with courage and diligence.

Bringing your awareness to your Crown chakra, imagine it radiating a soft, violet light. As your concentration deepens, visualize yourself becoming encapsulated in an orb of love and light. Allow any emotional pain and trauma that has been a part of your life to gently dissolve, allowing the vibrational force of spiritual love to enter. Each time you work with this visualization, be aware of any emotional ties that are holding you back, then hand these ties to the soft violet light to be transformed to a higher level of understanding.

STIMULATING ASANAS

The following yoga postures have been chosen because they work particularly on Sahasrara chakra. The head balance is a fairly advanced posture and should only be attempted once you are familiar with some of the more basic postures shown earlier in the book.

Expanded foot posture will benefit those unable to do the head balance. If you cannot touch the floor with your head, place a pile of books or a foam block between your legs to place your head on, resting your hands on your legs. As your inner thigh muscles become more supple, reduce the number of books.

On your first attempt, practise facing a wall in case you lose your balance. Hold this posture for as long as is comfortable, concentrating on a ray of violet light entering your Crown chakra. To return to the upright position, exhale, and on your next inhalation, raise the trunk of your body and bring your feet together.

When working with the head balance, you may initially like to practise with a chair (*as shown, right*) before attempting the full posture. It is known as 'the king of postures' and its mastery will give you poise and balance.

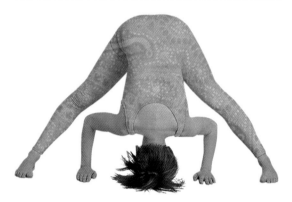

1 *Begin in standing posture (see page 15).*

2 *Inhale, moving your feet approximately one metre apart, keeping them level with one another.*

3 *On your next exhalation, with a straight spine, extend the trunk of your body forward from your hips, placing the palms of your hands on the ground with your fingers facing forwards.*

4 *Slowly walk your hands backwards until they are in line with your feet. At the same time extend the trunk of your body until the top of your head rests on the floor between your hands.*

5 *Hold your left ankle with your left hand and your right ankle with your right hand. Once you have acquired balance and are comfortable with this posture, bring your hands behind your back in the prayer position.*

BENEFITS:

This posture works on the inner thighs and hamstring muscles. It relieves stiffness in the shoulders and opens the chest. It increases blood flow to the neck, head and body.

SIRASANA
THE HEAD BALANCE

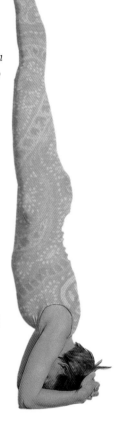

CAUTION:

People suffering from high blood pressure, neck problems, heart palpitations, thrombosis, chronic catarrh, chronic constipation, detached retinas or glaucoma should not practise this posture.

1 *Fold a blanket and place it on the floor in front of a wall. Kneel in front of the blanket and rest your forearms on the centre of it with your hands clasped and your elbows no further apart than your shoulders.*

2 *Place the crown of your head on the blanket between your cupped hands, so that the back of your head comes into contact with the palms of your hands. Straighten your legs, bringing your feet to the floor.*

3 *Slowly walk your feet towards your head until your thighs come into contact with your abdomen.*

4 *Lift up your spine, gradually taking the weight and balance of your body on to your arms and head. Slowly take your feet off the floor and when you feel securely balanced, straighten your legs.*

5 *When you are in the head balance, lift your body from the shoulders so that most of your body's weight is taken on your arms. There should be no pressure on your cervical spine.*

6 *Hold your concentration on your body, making minor adjustments to the posture where necessary. Initially, hold the posture for thirty seconds if you can. With practice, this time can be gradually increased until the posture can be held comfortably for thirty minutes.*

7 *When coming out of the head balance, slowly bend your knees and bring your feet down. Bend your knees and go into the child's pose (see page 15) and relax.*

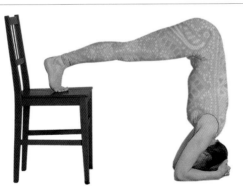

Another way of practising this posture is with a chair. Place the chair behind you, and instead of going into the full head balance, place your feet on the chair. Walk your feet forward on the chair until your spine is straight.

BENEFITS:

This posture increases the flow of blood to the brain, the pituitary and pineal glands. It rejuvenates the brain cells to make the brain function more efficiently and it increases vitality and sense of well-being. Because of the reverse flow of the blood, it is good for tired legs and varicose veins. It can also help prolapses of the bladder and uterus, relieve headaches and is beneficial for colds and asthma.

WORKING WITH THE YANTRA

The Crown chakra is symbolized by a thousand-petalled lotus, the number of completion, of total manifestation, and of infinity. When this chakra is fully open we become fully open to the light of the godhead. Our individual identity becomes lost as we merge with that ultimate reality. At this stage our emotional body has been dissolved, enabling us to see all creation with our inner sight. At this level, death holds no fear because there is no separation between self and spirit self. We recognize the physical body as the vehicle in which we live and know that death is but a discarding of this.

The shakti energy has awakened and risen through the Sushumna, opening and lifting the chakra's down-pointed heads to face the light of the spiritual sun. Shakti and Shiva have become unified in the Soma chakra and our duality has become transformed to wholeness.

A heightened state of awareness enables us to manifest and work with all forms of energy. We are now in command of the *siddhis*, or powers of yoga, but these fail to interest us because we realize that they can distract us from our now perfect state of being. We have become the master of our self and have the power to transmute energy into matter and matter into energy. We have become one with the divine and co-creator with it.

EXERCISE

Sitting comfortably, place the yantra where you are able to see it without straining your eyes. Start by moving your gaze around the outer part of the circle where the thousand petals of the lotus are formed. Contemplate the meaning of eternity, and how this relates to your own life. Search deep within yourself to discover how far you have travelled in your quest for your true self. Think about the eternal nature of your own soul and any fears you may have regarding the death of your physical body. Go still deeper into yourself and contemplate dying to self. This may be difficult unless you have experienced what you are dying to.

Dying to self is a state that necessitates detachment from all material possessions and emotional attachments to people, however close the relationship is with these souls. This does not mean that we stop loving them, but that we love them in a completely different way. One of the signs of spiritual growth is independence of external things. If we have true spiritual gifts, we maintain our independence from the things that surround us. The ten-

dency of the worldly mind is to look first to material comforts, but the wise make it their priority to establish themselves in spirituality. They never make the sacrifice of spirit to matter.

Moving your gaze to the inner circle with the full moon and sun, ponder upon the duality of nature and how you see yourself integrating your own duality to wholeness. The level of consciousness attained by the majority of the population necessitates the experience of duality. This means a need to experience the darkness in order to appreciate the light, to perceive the bad so that they can know what is good in their life. Most of us are still living in the sun's shadow but the age that we have now entered challenges us to walk forward into the full splendour and glory of the light.

Lastly, concentrate on the black circle at the centre of the yantra. This is the void where all the elements of the lower chakras have been refined to a state of beingness. We can only experience this state when we are still and silent. All wise people realize that the deeper part of their nature can only be expressed effectively when their mind and body are

still. That is why they often retire from the crowds and are not keen to offer their opinions. They think deeply and act quietly, knowing that it is in the moment of silence that the voice of the infinite is heard.

Shifting your concentration from the yantra to your physical body, quieten your mind and relax your body by concentrating

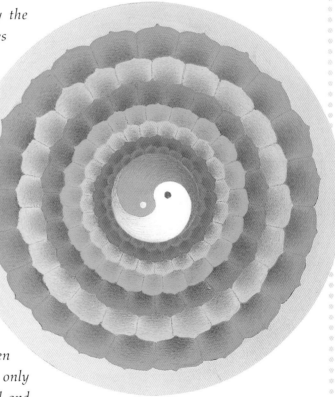

on the slow inhalation and exhalation of your breath. Then, listen; listen to the voice of the infinite within you.

OPENING THE CROWN CHAKRA THROUGH MEDITATION

The best way to open the Crown chakra is through meditation. This is the way to nourish the spirit and experience your inner world.

Meditation is commonly known to relax the mind and help to eliminate stress, but there is more to it than this. In yoga, meditation is described as a technique aimed to introvert the restless mind in order to gain knowledge of the higher self. The steps leading to this knowledge are introversion (*pratyahara*), concentration (*dharana*), meditation (*dhyana*) and, finally, transcendence (*samadhi*). These four steps are the last four of the eight steps of yoga laid down by the Eastern sage Patanjali.

There are many meditation techniques and it is worth trying as many of these as possible in order to discover the technique that works best for you. A technique advocated by many of the masters is meditating on the breath. This is favoured because the breath is always with us. Other methods use mantras, yantras, visualization and guided imagery, and further information on these may be sought from a qualified instructor.

Once you have discovered a technique that works for you, it is essential to practise for a period of time every day if you wish to make progress. Great insights do not happen overnight, sometimes it takes years of regular practice.

When meditating, one has to be detached from the meditation. Attachment involves the activity of the mind, therefore one cannot transcend it. If you are constantly looking for results, the very act of looking will prevent you from achieving them.

In his book *Meditations*, Krishnamurti, a great Eastern sage, explains: 'A meditative mind is silent. It is not the silence which thought can conceive of; it is not the silence of a still evening; it is the silence when thought – with all its images, words and perceptions – has entirely ceased. This meditative mind is the religious mind – the religion that is not touched by the church, the temples or by chants. The religious mind is the explosion of love. It is this love that knows no separation. To it, far is near. It is not the one or the many, but rather that state of love in which all division ceases. Like beauty, it is not of the measure of words. From this silence alone the meditative mind acts.'

A simple but very effective meditation technique can be done using a lighted candle. The candle's flame serves to remind us of our own inner light. Sit in a quiet place where

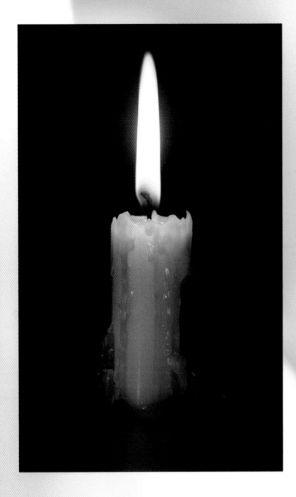

◀ *One of the most simple forms of meditation is performed using a lighted candle as your focus.*

tract your mind. Place a lighted candle where you can easily see it. Stare at the flame until your eyes start to tire. Then close your eyes and try to 'see' the flame of the candle in front of your closed eyes. When you see the flame it usually moves around and keeps disappearing. The aim is to keep it focused. When this flame finally disappears, open your eyes and again stare at the candle flame. Keep repeating this for twenty minutes.

Nothing is more glorious or potent than working with light. All the great masters have taught that the whole of our life is 'Maya', or illusion. The only way to pierce this veil is to recognize who we truly are, which takes many lifetimes of hard, disciplined work. Once this veil has been pierced, we see our inner light and recognize our divinity, and only then can we understand and answer the question 'Who am I?' with the answer 'I am that I am'.

May that light of unconditional love shine upon you and fill you with peace and understanding.

you will not be disturbed. If necessary, take the telephone off the hook. If you are anticipating the doorbell or the telephone ringing, you will be unable to practise meditation.

Sit comfortably on a chair or on the floor. If your body is not comfortable, it will dis-

125

Further Reading

Anodea, Judith, *Wheels of Life*, Llewellyn, 1999

Avalon, Arthur, *The Serpent Power*, Dover Publications, Inc., 1974

Gopi, Krishna, *The Secret of Yoga*, Turner Books 1973

Gopi, Krishna, *Kundalini – The*

Evolutionary Energy in Man, Shambhala 1985

Iyengar, Geeta S., *Yoga – A Gem for Woman*, Allied Publishers Private Ltd., 1983

Johari, Harish, *Chakras – Energy Centres of Transformation*, Destiny Books, 1987

Ozaniec, Naomi, *The Chakras*, Element, 1990

Singh, Jaideva, *The Yoga of Vibration and Divine Pulsation*, State University of New York Press, 1992

Index

Acknowledgements

PICTURE CREDITS
p.18 *Indira, the Ayran God of War, seated on an elephant*/Victoria & Albert Museum, London, UK/Bridgeman Art Library; p.22 Martial Colomb/Getty Images; p.24 Bob Krist/Corbis; p.38 EyeWire Collection/Getty Images; p.39 Inigo Jezierski/Getty Images; p.40 Akira Kaede/Getty Images; p.54 Siede Preis/Getty Images; p.56 James Gritz/Getty Images; p.70 Ryan McVay/Getty/Images; p.72 Akira Kaede/Getty Images; p.86 EyeWire Collection/Getty Images; p.88 Don Farrall/Getty Images; p.102 Oxford Scientific Films; p.125 (background) Skan/9/Getty Images; p.125 Photolink/Getty Images.

ADDITIONAL ILLUSTRATION CREDITS
Tsering Dorje; Anthony Duke; Harish Johari; J.B. Khanna and Co.

Illustrations by Harish Johari: *Chakras: Energy Centers of Transformation* by Harish Johari, Destiny Books, Rochester, VT 05767 USA, Copyright © 2000 by Pratibha Johari

Every effort has been made to acknowledge correctly and contact the source and/or copyright holder of each picture, and Eddison Sadd Editions apologises for any unintentional errors or omissions, which will be corrected in future editions of the book.

EDDISON•SADD EDITIONS

Commissioning Editor Liz Wheeler
Editor Nicola Hodgson
Proofreader Michele Turney
Indexer Dorothy Frame
Production Karyn Claridge, Charles James

Art Director Elaine Partington
Senior Art Editor Pritty Ramjee
Designer Malcolm Smythe
Picture Research Liz Eddison

Eddison Sadd Editions would like to thank Laura Knox for the specially commissioned photography and Susannah Marriott for modelling the yoga asanas.